Following Body Wisdom

How Energy Medicine Can Help Heal

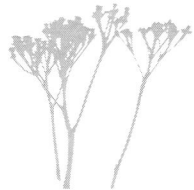

Atherton Drenth

Author's Note
All of the stories in this book are true. The names and identifying details have been changed to protect the client's privacy.
This book is not a substitute for medical help. If you are unsure if energy medicine can be of assistance, see your doctor. Energy medicine is not suitable for anyone undergoing extreme psychiatric distress or anyone who has been or is receiving medical assistance for extreme psychiatric distress.

Printed in Canada

ISBN 978-0-9813641-0-0

FIN 02 11 09

Library and Archives Canada Cataloguing in Publication

Drenth, Atherton, 1955-
        Following body wisdom : how energy medicine can help heal / Atherton Drenth.

ISBN 978-0-9813641-0-0

        1. Energy medicine. 2. Mental healing. I. Title.

RZ421.D74 2009   615.8'51   C2009-906410-3

For my husband
for always believing in me
and
my angels who guide me daily

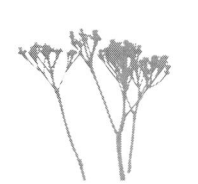

Contents

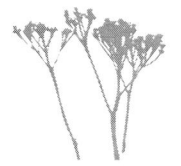

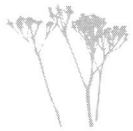

INTRODUCTION

If you are reading this then you have questions about energy medicine. You may be curious and wondering what on earth energy medicine is and if it is effective. You may also be wondering if this is something you want to try. It is my hope that this book will help to answer your questions.

I have been in private practice since 2000 and have personally conducted over 25,000 energy-healing sessions. Drawing from this vast well of experience, and being witness to so many miracles, I felt compelled to write about how energy work can be effective. In my experience a lot of new clients never come back after their first session because they don't understand what happened, or don't understand how to process what happened during their session. For the most part their reactions are skepticism and disbelief. How could something so simple, be so effective, so quickly?

It is my hope that this book will help to satisfy your curiosity or educate you about how energy medicine can be of service to you. I attempt to explain the principles of energy work, what to expect in a session, how to take care of yourself during a session and what you can expect after the session is over. I do this by sharing the personal stories of clients who have undergone major shifts in their lives as a result of this work. They have each graciously agreed to have their personal experiences put down on paper so that others can understand and benefit from them.

In my practice I see a growing trend where people feel like they are falling through the cracks of medical diagnosis. Most of these people have developed skepticism and distrust of the medical profession because it is no longer listening to what is happening to them as a patient and an individual. They are increasingly turning to energy work and other healing modalities as an alternative or adjunct to their allopathic medical treatments.

A client came in one day and said to me: "I don't know what you do and I don't care because it's helping and I feel better. I don't need a scientist to tell me what works for me." When I heard this, I was totally stunned. It was so true. Every client who uses energy work says something similar. They don't need anyone or any other system to tell them what to do. They are figuring it out for themselves and it is working. You will understand how this works as you read through this book.

My intent is to not tell you that energy medicine is the be all and end all. It isn't. It is NOT a substitute for allopathic medicine. But it is a modality that, if understood, can help. If, after reading this book, you feel that you want to give energy medicine a try, I *strongly* encourage you to seek out a practitioner in your area that exemplifies what has been outlined here. If you want to further educate yourself on what energy medicine has to offer, I refer you to the Suggested Reading page for a list of additional reading and study.

The body is very wise. It knows exactly what it needs and in what order it needs it. We just have to learn how to listen. Energy work does just that. It listens to what the body needs, teaches you how to understand its language and assists the body on its unique, healing journey. Energy work is self-empowering. May it be a guide to you on your own healing journey.

It is an honour to be of service.

Atherton Drenth
June 2009

"We are all born enlightened,
we are just not all conscious of our enlightenment"
Archangel Michael

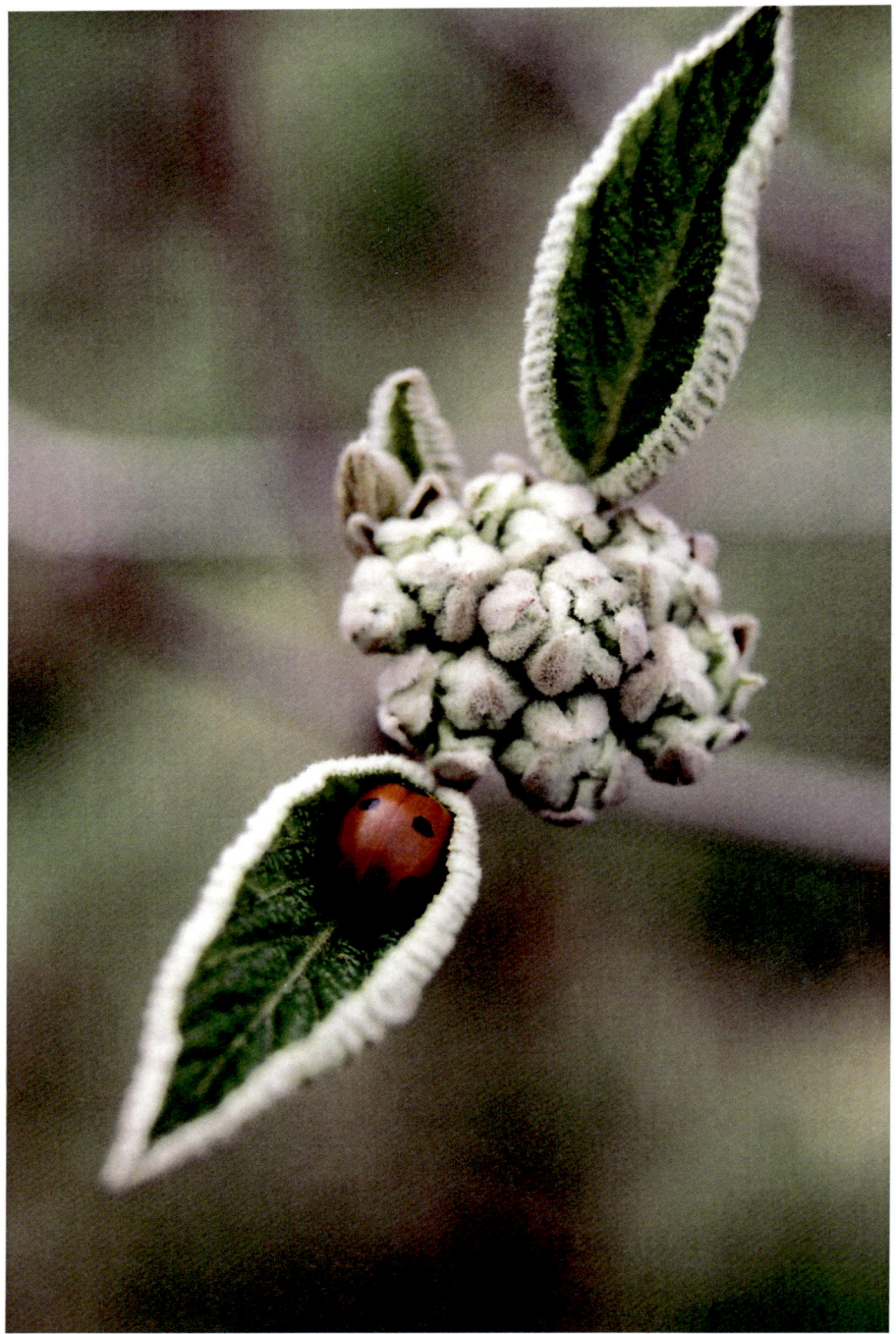

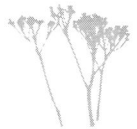

ENERGY WORK, ENERGY MEDICINE AND HEALING

The purpose of this book is to make energy work understandable and accessible to a broad audience. Not all *healers* are *energy workers* but all energy workers are healers. *Energy medicine practitioners* are often referred to as doing energy work or healing. For the purposes of this book I will use all three terms interchangeably. Practitioners of any of the above terms will also choose their own preference of how they want to be referred to. I see myself as a healer and an energy worker who practices energy medicine and therefore have chosen the term holistic energy therapist (HET) to describe what I do.

Many healers work with guides to assist in the healing journey. For example, I work with four archangels – Michael, Raphael, Ariel and Gabriel. I also work with Mother Mary and the Lord Jesus. They are present in the room with me in every session and hold safe and loving space for the client and for me. They will often offer profound insights to the client to assist them with their healing journey. I come from a Theosophical[1] Christian background. That is the basis of my spiritual life but I don't impose this belief system on my clients. My clients come from all different religious and spiritual backgrounds and we respect each other's beliefs.

Not all healers come from a religious or spiritual background and neither do their clients. I've worked with agnostics and atheists and get the

---

[1] See Glossary

same results. What's important is to understand that you don't need a religious or spiritual background to heal or help others to heal.

One of the most amazing things that my guides remind me of daily in my treatment room is:

> *"God is only love. There is no judgement. Judgement only comes from within yourself or it has come from another and you have decided to accept it as your own truth."*

For the purposes of this book I refer to God but readers can substitute spirit, the divine, source, universal consciousness or any other word that describes a higher power. I have a tendency to refer to God in the male gender even though I experience God as being "The All" – both male and female.

WHAT IS ENERGY WORK?

Energy work releases blocked energy that, if left unchecked, can eventually manifest in physical, emotional or spiritual symptoms. Most healers or energy workers can see energy fields, called auras, around all living things. They can examine auras in the client's field and see where the blocks are. They then work with the client to find out why the block is there and help them to release the blockage. That is energy work in a nutshell.

Energy work can be very subtle or it can be very dramatic. Sometimes it is so subtle that during a session you may not feel anything at all. At the end of the session you may have the impression that it was the "weirdest thing I have ever done in my life" yet in a day or two you suddenly notice that there has been a shift and you feel better somehow. Clients who have this experience make comments like: "I felt lighter, happier, more peaceful."

For some clients the session can result in feeling hot, cold, tingling all over, or they may feel their body is draining, releasing or that something is popping and letting go. The client can feel like their body is so heavy that they can't lift it off the table or they may feel so light they think they are going to float away. The sensations can also feel like gas moving through the abdomen or an organ can feel like it's quivering. Symptoms can also automatically change; for instance, pain stops, headaches disappear or cramping is no longer present. In the most dramatic cases clients begin to cry or feel angry and want to yell and thrash.

All of these reactions during and after a session are perfectly normal yet sometimes can be frightening because they have never been experienced before. The important thing is to understand that these are all normal indications that the energy is releasing and to allow the body to express this release. This is called *trusting the process*.

When I asked Archangel Michael what is the value of energy work he replied:

"Energy work brings the truth forward. People lose consciousness of why they are disturbed or upset. With energy work you assist them on their journey back through the layers of their energy (or memory) and help them and their body recall what created the block in the first place. This is not threatening, but a gentle unraveling of their own hurts, perceptions, realities and misnomers of what they themselves have conceived and presented to themselves as their truth. Where there is awareness, there is release and a healing miracle occurs."

We forget the body is a living, breathing organism. It feels. It feels through sensations. These sensations can be pleasure or pain. These sensations will "trigger" emotional responses in the mind. The body can only talk to you in symptoms or feelings. If you don't listen to it, eventually it will find another way to get your attention until finally you have a crisis. The crisis can be physical, emotional or spiritual. This is the point at which you will seek help.

ORDINARY MIRACLES

Every day in my healing practice I witness healing miracles. People are under the impression that miracles are dramatic earth shattering events. In some cases this is true but ordinary miracles do happen, every day. A miracle can be described as awareness of a simple truth. For example:

A person feels unloved. Yet one day they are walking down the street and a complete stranger smiles at them so radiantly that their heart almost hurts and it brings them to tears. They have experienced pure love from a stranger and their heart is opened. From this point forward they become open to loving experiences. Their fear that they are not loved has been challenged and forced to see the light. From this point forward the world takes on a different perspective because they have experienced love. They will now look for love in everything they see or do – this is a miracle.

> ### *Developing Gratitude*
>
> Every day find one thing in your life that you are grateful for. You will notice that if you continue this practice daily that your feelings of gratitude will expand to include two things, five things, 15 things until you realize that your day is filled with beauty and gratitude and it's hard to look upon the world with sadness and grief. This also becomes a miracle that everyone can experience in their lives

WHAT IS HEALING?

When we become sick we are looking to restore health and we want to be healed from our illness. To heal is described in the Oxford Dictionary as: "To become healthy again and to repair, correct (an undesirable condition, esp. a breach of relations); put right (differences etc.)." Health is described in the dictionary as: "The state of being well in body or mind."

WHAT IS A HEALER?

By my definition, a healer brings the physical body back into harmony with the energy body or aura and this manifests in the release of physical and emotional symptoms. Healers are guides and facilitators on each person's healing journey recognizing that the client is the expert. They see their role as a privilege and they are deeply honoured to be of service.

When I asked Mother Mary what is a healer, her response was:
"A healer is someone who helps another to heal."

Although there is no description in the Oxford Dictionary for "healer" they have been around since the dawn of man. Healers have gone by many names including shamans, medicine men or women, herbalists, midwives, intuitives etc. Regardless of their title, they are people who have a natural ability to understand energy (nature) and intuitively know how to assist in bringing the energy back into balance for the body or the tribe.

Every tribe has a healer. Every tribe knows their healers are connected to a wisdom that is beyond their daily reference of living. They trust this healing knowledge, believe it and practice it. They watch their children to see who demonstrates the natural abilities required of a healer. Once a child is identified as a potential healer, he or she apprentices with the tribe's healer who passes on the knowledge to the next generation. This ensures the tribes' survival and maintains a healing legacy.

Healers are intuitives who can see, sense, feel or hear energy fields or auras around all living things. A healer is a student of this energy and learns what the different patterns, colours and shifts mean. Healers learn how to clear stagnant or blocked energy in an aura by training in numerous modalities or remembering an innate knowledge. They just know how to heal without understanding the "why" or "what" of it and follow their instincts or intuition.

INTUITION

How we read and understand energy fields or auras is called intuition. Every human being has the ability to see or sense an aura, which means we are all born intuitive. We all have these intuitive abilities but have forgotten that we have them and tend to use them unconsciously. Mothers are often referred to as having "eyes in the back of their heads" because they often know if you are doing something you shouldn't. The stockbroker on Bay Street may be described as "having a good instinct" for business or stocks. The administrative assistant really "knows" his boss and is able to anticipate what is needed on any given day. Couples who have strong marriages will often be described as "being like two old shoes" and will finish each other's sentences in a conversation. The Myers-Briggs® Personality Assessments use Intuition as one of their markers. When we allow ourselves to remember our natural intuitive abilities it is called *developing your intuition.* There are numerous books, courses and exercises available to develop your intuitive abilities. I mention some of these in the glossary at the end of this book.

Not all healers see auras visually. Most healers perceive an aura or energy field in one of four ways based on what kind of intuitive they are:

- Clairvoyant
- Claircognizant
- Clairaudient
- Clairsentient

Clairvoyants "see" or perceive an aura or energy by using a chakra in their forehead called the third eye. This chakra allows them to view on an inner screen what they are perceiving at an energetic level. This chakra perceives subtle energy patterns and wavelengths. Information is received in clear pictures or impressions such as movies, colours or symbols.

Claircognizants "see" or perceive an aura through a knowingness[2]. They receive information through ideas or statements. Information is received as a complete idea. They know information, without knowing why they know. Claircognizants receive their information through their heart or crown chakras.

Clairaudients "hear" the information. The information can be heard as statements, sound, song, or vibration. Clairaudients receive their intuitive information through their ears.

Clairsentients "feel" the information in what are called body clues. They will feel the pain or discomfort in their own body and then be able to intuitively interpret why or where the pain is originating. Clairsentients receive most of their intuitive information through a chakra called the solar plexus but can "feel" that information anywhere in their bodies.

Healers, despite what type of intuitive they are, allow themselves to remember their natural abilities and then use them to help others to heal. A healer will see him or herself as a guide on each person's healing journey. They walk beside the client on their healing path. Healers never do anything the body can't handle or the mind won't accept. They understand that the body is very wise and knows exactly what it needs to do in order to heal. They trust the body to identify blockages or areas of stagnant energy that are ready to be released.

---

[2] Healers will often use the term knowingness to describe how they know something without understanding why they know it. The information is often received from a state of higher consciousness.

Once healers identify the blockage, they listen to why the block is there and help the client to release it in a safe, loving and non-judgemental environment. Healers understand that just because they know things about the client and can read their energy, they are not the expert on the client; the client is the expert. The body is also very wise and understands what it needs to heal. Healers can only read or see what the client wants or is ready to reveal. Healers can read energy fields and not minds.

HOLISTIC ENERGY THERAPISTS

Holistic Energy Therapists or HETs are intuitive healers and energy workers who practice energy medicine. They have been trained in numerous modalities such as Therapeutic Touch™ (TT), Biocomputer Operating System™ (B.O.S.), Total Body Modification™(TBM), and Reiki™ just to name a few. Many of them have been trained and certified as medical intuitives[3]. They use a blend of these modalities, as needed by the body wisdom, to assist in clearing blockages.

The body already knows how to heal itself but life gets in the way. A wound won't heal if it is infected. In the same way, the energy field can get blocked and needs assistance to release the blockage in order to heal or balance. There are a million different ways that the energy body can become blocked and they manifest on one of four levels:
- Physical
- Emotional
- Mental
- Spiritual

___
[3] See chapter on Training

Physical Level is influenced by poor diet, exposure to pollution, pesticides, chemicals, dehydration, physical wounding etc.

Emotional Level is influenced by how we respond to the world or how we perceive the world in response to us etc.

Mental Level is influenced by how we think about the world in relation to us etc.

Spiritual Level is influenced by allowing, misinterpreting or blocking connection to the divine.

The case histories cited later in this book are examples of these four different types of blockages and how energy work has assisted in clearing them so that the client could manifest healing.

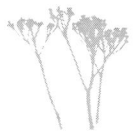

The Aura
The Energetic Body And Its Relationship To Healing

The human body is a physical form you can see, touch, feel and experience. It is a concrete form of energy that manifests as tissue (skin, hair, muscle, nerve, bone, blood, water, cells and DNA). We have developed ways of understanding this and have the science to back it up. Even though we are not intimately acquainted with how the human body looks on the inside, we trust science to tell us what it looks like and how it functions.

There is another form of the human body that is not concrete in our personal experience or realm of understanding. This is an energetic form that surrounds the physical body and is called the energy body or aura. Human beings have the most complex energy field or aura. The average human aura has an elliptical shape, radiates with different colours and extends out and around the body eight to 12 feet in all directions.

There are four major layers to the human aura – the physical, emotional, mental and spiritual. In a healthy human being the aura is egg shaped and radiates clear colours – every colour in the rainbow. This flow of energy and the colours of the aura change from moment to moment depending on thoughts, feelings and physical wellbeing.

The physical and the energy bodies flow and interact with each other naturally like our physical bodies do with the air around us. We are not conscious of the air around us but we know that it exists. We interact with air by breathing in oxygen and breathing out carbon dioxide. Plants breathe in carbon dioxide and breathe out oxygen. This symbiotic relationship benefits both us and our natural environment.

The layers of our aura interact with each other and the physical body in a similar way – there is a symbiotic relationship that is beneficial to every layer. When the body is healthy we call that *being in energetic harmony* or *balance*. When any aspect of the physical body or energy body is out of balance, there will be a manifestation of symptoms. At a physical level, the symptoms can manifest as pain; at an emotional level, depression; at a mental level, a recurring thought (i.e. nobody likes me) and at a spiritual level it can manifest as a loss of purpose.

The purpose of energy work is to bring all the layers of the aura back into balance so there is a harmonic symbiotic relationship between the physical and energetic layers. Holistic energy therapists (HETs) or healers work with disruptions in the energy body and release them. This allows the physical body to harmonize which manifests as good health.

For example, at the spiritual level you have rediscovered your purpose, at the mental level you know that you are loved and accepted, at the emotional level you are happy and joyful and at the physical level you are pain free.

How do we prove that the aura really exists? Scientists and the medical community tell us that auras do not exist because in their realm of science there are no definitive tools that measure them. They cannot see the energy body with their physical eyes. Despite this fact they are already measuring aspects of the physical energy field using instrumentation such as the electrocardiogram (ECG) which measures electrical currents from the heart; the electroencephalogram (EEG) which measures electrical currents from the brain and lie detectors which measure electropotential of the skin. But because they cannot "see an aura" with their physical eyes or definitively prove that auras exist scientifically, they assume that anyone who does believe in them, or says they can "see" them must be delusional. Yet in the last 60 years instrumentation has been developed that is beginning to change that perspective.

In the late 1930s, Russian scientists Semyon Kirlian and his wife, Valentina, discovered a technique of taking pictures of the auric field by directing a high frequency electrical field at an object. It is called Kirlian Photography.

Based on this work and other research, Russian physicist Dr. Konstantin Korotkov developed an instrument that records electro-photonic images and calls this technique Gas Distribution Visualization or GDV.

Cyndi Dale, in her book, *The Subtle Body* states: "It is known that biofields exist because they have been imaged with newer technology, including Kirlian photography, aura imaging and Gas Discharge Visualization."[4] These new technologies are beginning to generate a lot of interest in some scientific circles.

As a result, scientific and medical communities are very slowly beginning to acknowledge that auras might possibly exist and that they can

---

[4] Dale, Cyndi. The Subtle Body: An Encyclopedia of Your Energetic Anatomy. Sounds True Publishing. Boulder Colorado 2009.

provide clues to the nature of illness – something that healers have known for millennia.

Let us not forget that until the invention of the microscope the scientific and medical communities did not believe in bacteria. The human race also believed that the world was flat until Columbus sailed to the Americas. The bottom line; just because you can't see it, doesn't mean that it doesn't exist.

In actual fact, everyone can see auras. We are all born with the ability to see auras but we usually lose consciousness of this ability as small children. And yes, small children under the age of two generally do see auras but they learn very quickly that others around them don't so they shut it down. Let me give you an example.

We have all had the experience of holding a newborn in our arms. We gaze down at the baby and are amazed at this little tiny human being. We are amused at how the newborn moves its eyes around but have been led to believe the baby cannot focus on an image and see detail. If you watch carefully however, you will begin to notice that the baby's eyes seem to focus on the area above your head instead of on your face. What the baby is actually looking at is the energetic eminence from the top of your head, which is usually the brightest part of an aura. A doctor will tell you that the baby cannot see anything more than shapes and movement. Bingo. That is what an aura is. An aura looks like a misty cloud of energy around the physical body; it flows in shapes and movements like a fog.

Now fast forward to this little baby being two years old. The child is beginning to discover drawing. The mother eagerly gives the child paper and crayons and asks the child to draw what it sees. The child may look around and start to draw large circles or vague shapes. The mother in her enthusiasm will say, "Let's draw a tree". The child looks at the tree and picks up a purple crayon and again draws a fuzzy shape. The mother, thinking she is helping her child to develop says, "Oh, this is how you draw a tree. This is a brown crayon and the trunks are brown." The child suddenly realizes that Mom "sees" the world differently and "learns" how to see the world the way the parent does because they want to be accepted.

The education system will then reinforce this behaviour of what each colour is and what it represents. The child has to conform in order to be accepted and to get good marks at school and now believes that trees are brown and green and can no longer perceive trees energetically. It is as simple as that.

Shamans and healers have known for thousands of years that auras do exist because they know how to perceive or "see" the aura.

How do healers see or perceive auras? They see the aura using what in eastern spiritual traditions is called the third eye, which is located in the middle of the forehead. When you choose to train as a healer, your third eye is reopened and you learn to discern the different energy patterns and what they mean for the body and client.

In essence this means there are two different ways of seeing – one is the physical act of seeing and the other is the energetic form of seeing. Healers can see the physical body and they can also shift their gaze to see the body energetically. The easiest way to illustrate this shift in gaze is using the Magic Eye®[5] or 3D images as an example. Most people have seen computer-generated images that at first look like one thing and then when you shift your gaze to soft focus, you see the hidden 3D illusion. In the same way healers will shift their eyes from 3D sight to soft gaze and be able to see the aura and its colours.

---

[5] For more information on and materials on Magic Eye® contact: www.magiceye.com

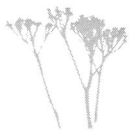

THE PROCESS OF HEALING
A NEW PARADIGM

The process of healing is undergoing a major shift in public understanding and awareness. People are finding that working solely within a medical model that focuses on specific symptoms, is not working. Too many people find themselves falling between the cracks, or stuck on a merry-go-round of medical professionals, therapies and medications while improved health still eludes them. Repeatedly I hear from clients: "There has to be more than this. There has to be another way." Maybe it's time to take a look at the process of healing from within a different paradigm.

This *new healing paradigm*[6] implies that we need to look at the body as a whole instead of just looking at the symptoms of illness. This shift creates a process of self-empowerment or accepting your own inner authority. Eastern philosophy teaches that we are not just our bodies — we are energy. Quantum physics[7] teaches us that we are a very complex system of energetic patterns. We are learning that we cannot isolate one thing from a complex pattern without creating an impact on the whole system. A symptom does not necessarily signify one specific problem, but rather that something is out of balance within the whole body.

Our current medical model has relied heavily on isolating and treating symptoms. It is an illness-based, rather than a wellness based model of

---

[6] See Glossary
[7] See Glossary

how we view our health. We are learning that each person is truly an individual and how one person responds to an illness will not necessarily result in the exact same pattern in another. This is because the whole system is affected by its physical and emotional history. When we are working within an illness-based model, we rely on common symptoms as opposed to honouring how the symptoms manifest in the individual. In this model, we learn to accept the authority of the medical community because they are the recognized experts on symptoms and how to deal with them.

 We have been trained to accept outside authority – anyone who has more education or is a so-called "expert" has authority over us.

We make the assumption that other people know us better than we know ourselves and therefore know what's right for us. Currently in the developed world, health and healing is conducted in a medical model that I refer to as the *patriarchal medical model*[8] This model follows a chain of command. For example:

You are suffering from constipation and migraines and you go to your family doctor, who prescribes medication for the migraines and tells you to improve your diet. The side effects of the medication cause constipation and so you go back to the family doctor to say that now the constipation is even worse. She tells you to drink more water and increase the fiber in your diet. Then you start suffering from acid reflux, bloating and you start to break out in hives. The constipation continues to be an issue so now your doctor gives you a laxative. Laxatives aren't

---

[8] Symptom based healing model; treating symptoms. (Author's definition).

helping so the doctor refers you to a specialist who deals with gastrointestinal (GI) issues. The GI specialist says that you need to take medication for the acid reflux and prescribes medication that creates the side effect of constipation. So now you're on medication for migraines, you're afraid to eat, you're constipated and your migraines become so debilitating that you're having to take time off work. You go back to the doctor and she decides that maybe it's a psychosomatic issue and sends you to see a psychiatrist. The psychiatrist tells you that you're suffering from borderline depression and you need to take an antidepressant – the side effects of this medication being weight gain, bloating and constipation. You begin to suffer from heart palpitations and you pass out at work. You're rushed into the emergency department and the cardiac specialist that sees you says that you're suffering from anxiety and stress and that you need to go back to your psychiatrist and have your meds changed. Finally one day you can't work, you can't go to the bathroom and you realize that something is horribly wrong. You go back to your family physician and demand that more extensive tests be done. She finally decides to send you for a barium test and the radiologist discovers a mass in your abdomen and requests a biopsy of the small intestine. Finally, they discover that you're an undiagnosed person with celiac disease.

This is the patriarchal model of medicine that looks to resolve the symptoms without looking for the cause. It also views medical practitioners as being the experts on their clients and their health. Energy medicine on the other hand, is based on what I call a *matriarchal healing model*[9] that looks for the cause to heal the symptoms. It acknowledges that clients are the experts on their own body and health

---

[9] Looking at the body as a whole, at all levels, energetically. (Author's definition)

because they know what they feel. The matriarchal model works from the whole body system. It acknowledges that the client's body wisdom knows what exactly is causing the symptoms. If you remove the cause of the symptoms, the body will heal itself.

Let's go back to the scenario described earlier and how it would be handled by energy medicine.

A client suffers from migraines and constipation. The HET connects to the body and asks the body to show the cause of the migraines. The body reveals deep-seated resentment and anger. When these emotions are tracked through the body it is found that these emotions are centered in and around the small intestine. When the practitioner goes to the small intestine, these repeated statements are heard from the body: *I am in pain. This hurts*. When the body is asked to clarify the cause of the pain it is revealed that the client has food allergies. The practitioner investigates through the body what the body is reacting to and discovers sensitivities to wheat and gluten. The practitioner refers the client to their family physician for a blood test for celiac disease and the test confirms what the body has been saying all along, it has an allergy to gluten (celiac disease).

In this model the practitioner is working with the whole body in partnership with the client and the doctor. The practitioner is the not the expert on the client but is trained how to hear the whole body and then teaches the client how to honour what they are hearing.

For example, as a child this client suffered from constant bellyaches. Her parents insisted that she finish everything on her plate despite the fact that she was complaining that her stomach hurt when she ate. She learned to silence that bellyache or inner pain and do as she was told because her parents were the authority. Over time, she became resentful of her parents and felt that they didn't understand her. As an adult, this resentment began to manifest as migraines. When she was diagnosed as having celiac disease, and made the appropriate dietary changes, all of her digestive issues cleared and she was then free to unravel the feelings of anger and resentment that had developed in her childhood with her therapist.

This way of healing is a new paradigm because it no longer focuses on the symptoms but looks at the cause that is revealed in the body. And when you uncover a cause, you are responding to whole-body healing. An energy medicine practitioner or holistic energy therapist (HET) is trained to listen and help the client interpret what's really going on. The body's only language is symptoms and we have lost the art of listening to those symptoms as a whole and recognizing that they are cries for help.

An energy medicine practitioner or a HET recognizes and ensures that the client is aware that they are their own expert and the practitioner is there to assist and interpret, always making sure that what is being stated feels true to the client. Compare this to an interpreter who understands sign language and translates on behalf of the person who is hearing impaired.

Energy medicine is not for the faint of heart – it forces you to take a look inward at what you are feeling, on a physical or emotional level and this is not always a comfortable process. This is because we are not generally encouraged to be emotional as the people around us can't bear to see us in emotional pain. They expect us to be just fine. But when we give ourselves permission to undertake this healing journey we enter into a process of discovery, understanding, and most importantly we lovingly give ourselves permission to explore and allow change.

It is not considered socially acceptable to feel and express our emotions. Feeling sick or emotional all the time? Your symptoms must be psychosomatic and you need to take antidepressants to stabilize your emotions. Can't cope with life? Get a therapist. Having a problem in your life? It must be your partner, your job or your relationship with your parents.

If you try to talk about your problems with others the usual responses are:

"How can you feel that way when there are so many people suffering in the world?"

"Who are you to complain?"

"You think you've got problems, wait until you hear what's going on with me."

We are not allowed the freedom to experience and express our inner self. We are encouraged by society and its current belief systems to be strangers to our own bodies and feelings.

Energy medicine offers the opportunity to go back and heal what was left wounded. It is a gentle loving process. It offers the opportunity to see yourself with deeper compassion and love. It often results in profound, lasting healing and a new understanding of who you are. This is called *self-empowerment*.

For the majority of clients who try energy medicine, it is often their last resort; they have tried everything to resolve their symptoms and have found no relief. Many clients come with a healthy dose of skepticism but they very quickly start to notice positive results and become advocates for energy medicine. Some clients find the process too different and are afraid to take responsibility for their health and make the changes necessary. Or, they need scientific proof about why it does work, in order to feel safe trying it. Energy medicine is not for everyone.

This new paradigm of healing called energy medicine is here to work in cooperation with all healing modalities, traditional or complementary, because energy medicine works with the whole. This process of healing is the true meaning of *holistic health*.

HETs are not a substitute for a doctor or allopathic[10] medical care. We are very fortunate to have the health-care system that we do in Canada and our doctors provide a level of care that is unprecedented world-wide. HETs don't need to replace what is already working but it is our hope that we will be able to demonstrate to existing medical models that there is another way to help our clients heal.

We are open to working in harmony with existing allopathic medical practitioners. There are medical doctors that are open to working in

---

[10] Allopathic is another term for conventional or traditional medicine. See Glossary

conjunction with HET and energy medicine because they have noticed that their patients are healing more quickly. We are confident that energy medicine, working in conjunction with allopathic medicine, will be the new paradigm of healing for the future.

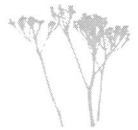

Embarking on a Healing Journey
The Matriarchal Healing Wheel

In the beginning when I posed the question to my angel guides, "How do you build a *healing team*?" I was shown an image of a wagon wheel. The angels called this a *"Healing Wheel"* and told me that the hub in the middle represents the individual. They told me that each spoke of the wheel represents a healing practitioner (alternative or traditional) and they further explained that each spoke added to the wheel gives it additional strength and provides momentum. The individual or client is the hub – they decide what is to be included inside the wheel and how the wheel will move forward. In other words, the client decides which practitioners they want to work with and how they want to work with them.

When a person discovers that they have a health issue, they need to decide how they are going to deal with that and who they are going to work with. By choosing which practitioners they wish to work with, and how they want their course of treatment to go, they are building their own personal healing team and embarking on their healing journey.

The Angels explained that a healing journey is a journey of awareness and experience that helps a person who is unwell find their path to wellness. This is where the healing journey becomes not only about overcoming physical symptoms, but also the mental attitudes and beliefs, as well as the emotional and spiritual experiences, that may have contributed to the illness.

Undertaking a healing journey is nothing new or extraordinary – most people have already embarked on a healing journey at one time or another. For example, if a person comes down with the flu she embarks on a healing journey (becomes her own healing team) and looks after herself by resting and drinking lots of fluids. In this example there does not immediately appear to be an underlying emotional, mental or spiritual cause for her illness but upon further reflection these causes may appear. She may not understand that she has become ill because she has not been taking care of her body. She has been ignoring the fact that she has not been getting enough sleep and has been pushing through her fatigue. She has been suppressing feelings of unhappiness with her job and her career. As a result, she has been feeling unhappy and consequently eating poorly. This puts a lot of strain not only on the immune system – the engine of the body – but also on the emotional and mental bodies creating more fatigue. The body will often choose something simple, like a flu or cold, to force the emotional or mental body into a state of rest and reflection.

While she has the flu, she may realize that it is time to take a look at her lifestyle. Perhaps she might realize how unhappy she is with her life and take action. She might begin to prioritize her commitments, realign her career goals and treat her body with more respect. She might decide to get more rest, drink lots of fresh water and add more healthful foods to her diet.

Another example of embarking on a healing journey is a person who suffers whiplash following a car accident. He may choose to see a doctor, physiotherapist, a chiropractor and a holistic energy therapist for energy work. He has just created his own healing wheel. For his journey he seeks each practitioner's advice and decides on a prescribed course of treatment which feels right to him. It may include energy work, massage, exercise, chiropractic adjustments and follow-up appointments with his doctor.

In this case, how could a car accident resulting in a whiplash injury be anything more than a physical event? Is there a possibility that there is an emotional or spiritual layer that influenced this accident?

Through his energy work he discovers that he believes that "nothing in life ever goes right." Because of this underlying belief system, the universe has no option but to honour his free will and a car accident can be an outcome. During the course of his recovery from the whiplash, and further energy work, he may uncover this repeating pattern of negative belief that has influenced the course of his entire life. He is now in a position to consciously choose to change this negative belief. This unfortunate event then becomes a catalyst to create a change in perception in how he views his life and the world. He may begin to realize that he has never been able to stay in a long-term relationship because he's afraid that "things are never going to go right" so he is always looking for the flaws and waiting for something to go wrong. He may also realize that he never really liked the car anyway and was wishing that he could get a new one.

He now decides to change that core negative belief to a positive one such as, "my life is joyful and successful". The end result in this change of belief is that he is finally able to go into a relationship without fear.

Years later he may look back at this car accident and realize that it was a positive turning point in his life. It gave him the opportunity that he needed to change his belief system and heal his life – physically, emotionally and spiritually.

HEALING TEAM

A healing team can consist of any types of healing professionals – traditional or complementary. It can be any number of practitioners: physician, chiropractor, homeopath, naturopath, psychotherapist, dentist, clinical aromatherapist, massage therapist and a holistic energy therapist. The individual decides who is on their healing team. They will make these decisions based on personal choice, expertise and specialty. All of these practitioners then become spokes on the client's personal healing wheel. What is important to understand here is that the individual is the centre of the wheel and they decide who they will choose to be on their healing team. This is the new paradigm – a new model of healing, also called the matriarchal model. The client chooses the best course of healing based on what they know to be right for them, personally.

HOW TO BUILD YOUR OWN HEALING TEAM

Always remember YOU are your own expert. No one knows you better than you. I am often surprised that when I remind clients of this they look startled. Most of them have never looked at their own bodies and life that way. We have become accustomed to allowing someone else to always be the expert. We have given away our power and have lost the ability to decide what is right for ourselves based on how we feel.

I personally had to face this loss of power with my own health struggle; for years I tried to find answers as to why I was having so many health problems. "There is nothing wrong with you," was all I ever heard from the medical community. They would tell me that if I took this drug I would be fine – it made me more ill. If I exercised more I would be fine – it made me more ill. If I saw a therapist I would be fine – I cried my heart out and didn't get better. Everyone I consulted was analyzing my symptoms but when I finally went to a healer, he taught me to listen to my body and my feelings. For the first time I was able to discover the cause of my symptoms and find my path to healing.

The exception to this rule is for small children. For parents of small children I always say: "You are the only advocate your child has." For mothers especially, they need to remember that they carried that baby around inside them for nine months. No one knows or understands that child's needs better than you do. And for parents who adopt a child, the same principle applies. Because you have wanted that child for so long that when you finally hold that child in your arms there is an instant attachment and within weeks you begin to understand how to read *your child*. Don't ever discount that intuitive wisdom.

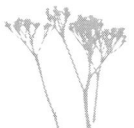

GUIDELINES
CHOOSING YOUR OWN COMPLEMENTARY HEALTH CARE TEAM

- Selecting Your Own Health Care Team – Who Do You Choose?
- Personal Referrals - Ask Your Friends
- The First Meeting – What To Ask
- Be Selective – What You See Is What You Get
- Keep Your Own Records – It's Your Health Care

SELECTING YOUR OWN HEALTH CARE TEAM – WHO DO YOU CHOOSE?

Any practitioner, whether they be traditional or complementary can be part of your health care team. You already have a team in place; you may not be aware of it or call it that. For example, a typical traditional health care team may consist of:

- Physician
- Massage Therapist
- Personal Trainer
- Dentist
- Physiotherapist
- Life Coach
- Pediatrician
- Therapist
- Chiropractor

To build on a typical traditional health care team you would incorporate elements from complementary therapies.

Here is an example of a health care team using both traditional and complementary modalities. This illustrates that you can combine elements from both healing streams for your health care team.

NEW PARADIGM - HEALTH CARE TEAM

TRADITIONAL	COMPLEMENTARY
• Physician	• Naturopath
• Dentist	• Medical Intuitive
• Pediatrician	• Cranial Sacral Therapist
• Specialist	• Holistic Allergist
• Massage Therapist	• EFT[11] Practitioner
• Physiotherapist	• Medical Intuitive
• Psychotherapist	• Homeopath
• Personal Trainer	• Clinical Aromatherapist
• Life Coach	• Reflexologist
• Osteopath	• Yoga Instructor
• Chiropractor	• Holistic Energy Therapist

PERSONAL REFERRALS - ASK YOUR FRIENDS

Personal referrals are usually the most reliable form of finding a competent complementary health care provider. Ask around, talk to people. Who do they see? What do they like about them? If someone is practicing a modality you are unfamiliar with, go to the Internet and read up on the modality. Call the practitioner's office and ask them send you more information. The library can be a terrific resource for additional material.

---

[11] See Glossary

THE FIRST MEETING – WHAT TO ASK

- How long have you been practicing?
- Are you trained in other healing modalities? If so, what are they and how do you decide what to use? (*Muscle testing*[12] is the most accurate determination)
- Do you work in person, *distance*[13] or over the phone?
- Do you refer? If so, how do you decide when to refer?
- What other health care professionals do you work with?
- What did you do before you became a healer?
- Why did you become a healer?
- How did you become a healer?
- How do you feel about my working with other practitioners?
- Who is on your healing team?
- How do you take care of your own health?

Come prepared to your first appointment. Bring your complete health history and copies of any medical reports that you have. If you find that what they have to offer is not what you are looking for don't stop looking just because one practitioner or modality isn't able help you. With complementary health care, if you wrote down all of your issues, symptoms and history and took that information to ten different health practitioners, there would be ten different interpretations and recommendations for help. Take notes and see what pieces feel right to you.

If the complementary health care practitioner makes you feel inferior, ignorant, or tells you that you can only work with them – leave. A healing wheel is a team effort. In my experience complementary health care

---

[12] See Glossary
[13] See Glossary

providers are very open to working with any member of your healing team. But always remember you have choice and you are doing the choosing.

BE SELECTIVE – WHAT YOU SEE IS WHAT YOU GET

Over the years I have learned that "what you see is what you get." I have learned to trust my intuition and read not only the practitioner but also the environment in which they work. When I am choosing a professional for my health care team I use these as my personal guidelines. How do they present themselves? Are they nicely dressed? Are they professional?

- Does their environment feel comfortable and safe to you?

- How is their office organized? Is it clean? As a former office manager I know someone is having trouble with their business if they can't keep a clean office.

- How do they answer the phone? Does their voicemail message sound professional? Is it clear? It is amazing how quickly you can find out about a professional by the way they answer and talk on the phone or how their voicemail is recorded.

- Do they have any information on the Web, brochures or business cards? Is the information clear, concise? How does it make you feel when you read it? If their website and brochure are confusing, does this mean they aren't clear about what they do?

- What are their credentials? Look around their treatment room or front office. Are their qualifications posted? If not, ask them about their training.

- Do they answer questions easily? Watch their body language. How do they make you feel when you ask questions?

- Do they look healthy? Who looks after them? If a practitioner tells me that they are their own health care team, I leave. If they can't trust other practitioners then they will be reluctant to refer out when they are at their limit of competence. If they are reluctant to refer or say that they prefer that you work only with them – leave.

- Ask them how they came to be a complementary health care professional. The stories may surprise you and will probably give you a sense of who the practitioner is and if they are a good fit for you.
- Be aware that helping professionals, regardless of their training and expertise, are human beings. Never put them on a pedestal and be wary of a practitioner who expects to be treated like they should be on a pedestal. Remember you are interviewing them for your healing team because you are the expert on you.

Every discipline has been created over time and each has its own unique history, philosophy, frame of reference, techniques, and style. This history and their training shape the way a practitioner sees and deals with you. If you find that the tools they use are unfamiliar or complex and it is confusing and making you feel intimidated, ask more questions. Complementary health care providers should be happy to answer all your questions.

KEEP YOUR OWN RECORDS – IT'S YOUR HEALTH CARE

Keep a copy of all your medical records, tests, scans etc. Carry them with you and don't be afraid to ask for copies of your records. Remember this is your healing journey. Keep a journal of your visits – who you saw, date, what was recommended and how you processed after the session. The more complete the information, the better you are at being the expert on you.

PROFESSIONAL ETHICS

I would like to say a few words about professional ethics. Healers and energy medicine practitioners have been around since the dawn of mankind and as mentioned earlier, they have been called by many different names. They have been referred to as shaman, healer, midwife, herbalist, medicine man, etc. and have sometimes been vilified and persecuted by society. The scientific community still has difficulty understanding what it is that energy healers do. As a result we have had to work quietly in the background and over the years developed our own code of professional ethics. Some of us belong to associations, others do not. But the practitioners I have chosen to work with have always displayed a high degree of professionalism. Lori Wilson [14] has done a beautiful job in her book, *"de-mystifying Medical Intuition"*, so I will quote her standards for ethical boundaries, taught by her association:

Practitioners who have clear ethical boundaries state what they can and cannot do, or will or will not do, according to their own personal style of work and ethical standards

---

[14] Re-printed with permission: de-mystifying...Medical Intuition. Lori Wilson Education Corporation. 2005.

- They are not swayed by emotions of well-meaning relatives or curious friends

- They will not talk about clients in social settings

- If they do ask colleagues for support or consultation, they will never include their client's name and it will always be with the express verbal consent of their client

- Practitioners with clear boundaries will always ensure that clients have given their consent for intuitive services, if they are asked to work in conjunction with other health professionals as a resource, or they are using the outside consultations to further their own learning

THE BOTTOM LINE

Coming from a medical technology background, and also as a former business manager, I have very strong personal opinions about how complementary health care professionals should present themselves.

I was raised in a family business and my father taught us that if you want credibility, you live it, work it and produce it. In other words he was teaching: "If you are going to talk the talk, walk the walk". He always believed that what you see is what you get. I believe he was right. When embarking on a healing journey remember:

- You are your own expert

- Trust your intuition

- Believe in yourself

- Look at what you are getting and ask yourself "Is this right for me?"
- Never be afraid to leave if it doesn't feel right
- You always have a choice

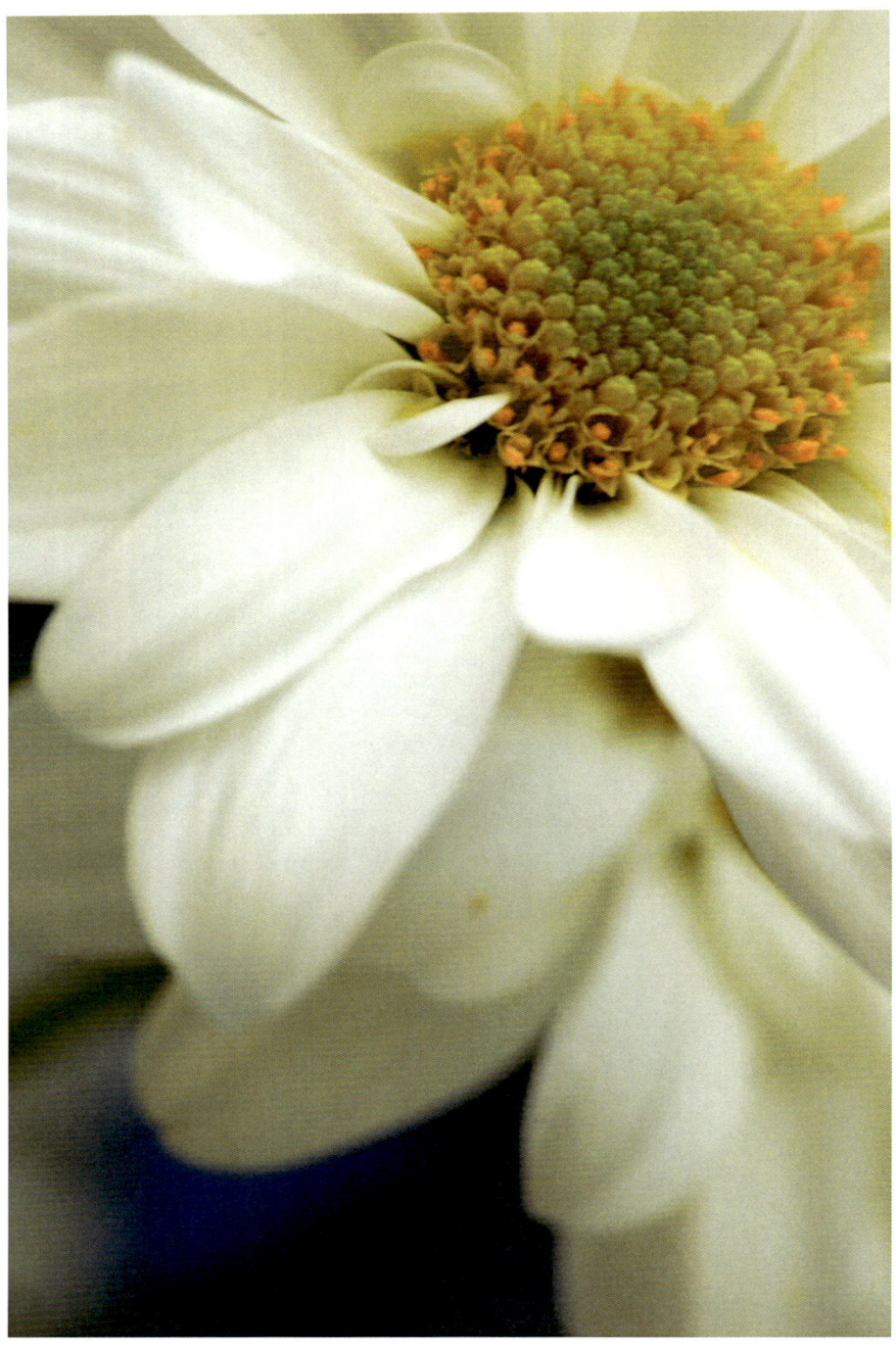

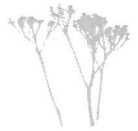

My Personal Journey
THE BIRTH OF A HEALER

My earliest childhood memories are of angels. They intervened on my behalf and their voices gave me guidance that kept me safe. I remember lying in bed at night watching spirit lights in my bedroom until I fell asleep and having visions that foretold my future. There was one grand-fatherly voice in particular that was always present giving me advice and comfort.

As a child I was raised in a rather eclectic, eccentric family environment where both of my parents had psychic abilities so what I was experiencing was considered normal. I never really questioned it. As I was growing up however, I needed to learn when to speak and when not to speak.

I remember when I was about five years old I was in my father's printing shop and he was talking to a customer. I instinctively knew that this customer was lying to my father and told him that. My father just shook his head to keep me quiet and so I said it again. "Daddy, he's lying to you." Again my father shook his head and told me to go into the back of the shop. Later after the customer was gone, my father came to me and said, "Atherton, I knew he was lying to me but sometimes you just got to know when to hold it (the truth you know inside) and when to say it." This has been a very difficult lesson for me to learn.

As a teenager I never really fit in and was considered "odd" by my peers. I developed a bad habit of blurting things out because I had visions about things happening to my friends and they didn't always appreciate my "advice". For example, I instinctively knew that one of the "popular" girls in my class was going to get into trouble with her boyfriend if she didn't go on the pill. I suggested that she go on the pill and she looked at me like I was totally weird. Good girls at that time didn't fool around like that. She was shocked and so were all of us when she got pregnant six months later. This kind of behaviour made me less than popular and I often ate my lunch alone. High school would have been a very lonely time had I not had such a rich inner life.

During these early years I was doing a lot of reading about psychic phenomena and spirituality. My mother coached me through Theosophy[15] and I began practicing meditation.

From very early on I believed that people could heal others but they either had to be a holy person, like a saint, or were born with full awareness of their healing ability. My mother, for example, was reading people's palms in her community by the time she was five. I would then read stories about people who saw "auras" and I wondered why I couldn't see them. It didn't matter how hard I tried, I could not see them. Even so, I spent a lot of time thinking about the ability to do healing work. Never did I think or dream that it was possible to awaken sacred knowledge from within and that one day I would become a healer.

As an adult in the workforce I couldn't understand why my colleagues would tell me that I was intuitive and that I sometimes scared them. In

---

[15] See Glossary

the lunchroom I would blurt things out without meaning to. Once I asked a colleague how her baby was doing. She said the baby was just fine and I said, "Oh," with surprise. She asked me why I wanted to know and I said, "I just wanted to make sure that the baby was OK." The next day we found out that she'd spent the night in the hospital with the baby who had suddenly run a high fever and had a seizure. Thankfully the baby was OK.

Over time I developed a reputation and co-workers found me unnerving. When I became a manager, I had an uncanny ability to see how projects were going to turn out if certain things didn't happen. My bosses would find this threatening and would tell me to "cool it" because I was intimidating the staff. Working for others became a very confusing and unhappy time in my life.

My very first memory of healing occurred when I was about four years old. My father's business was in trouble and my mother wanted to protect us in case he went bankrupt so she sent my sister Althea and I away for the summer to a farm. One day we were playing in a part of the barn with lots of old tools and cats. My sister stepped on a board with a rusty nail that went right through her shoe into her foot. Naturally, the farmer's wife took her to the hospital. Althea screamed when they gave her a shot for tetanus. I remember looking at the needle and going into shock. As far as I was concerned that needle might as well have been 10 feet long and every inch of it seemed to disappear into her skinny little leg. The whole experience terrified me.

The next morning, I was playing in the same shed and stepped on the same nail and hurt myself, exactly the same way. I pulled the nail from my foot and snuck into the summer kitchen and quietly washed my foot but was caught by the farmer's wife. She was furious. She demanded to know what had happened and wanted an explanation for my being in the house. In my fear I vehemently denied everything and hid the angry, red puncture hole on the bottom of my foot. As punishment for being in the house, I was sent to my room without dinner. I remember looking at the hole in my foot and saying to myself, "This has got to be gone in the morning." I quickly fell asleep. The next morning when I woke up and looked at my foot, the nail hole was completely gone. There was not even a scar or trace of the puncture wound. The joy I felt was pure ecstasy. I had gotten away with it and didn't need to have that terrible needle. I remember thinking, "Oh, I can heal myself."

My next clear memory of healing occurred when I was about 14 years old. Our family raised Siamese cats, and they quickly became a personal passion. By this stage of my life I wanted to become a veterinarian and got a part-time job working for a local vet clinic. Our neighbors also had a Siamese cat and she was pregnant. It became my mission to ensure that she was properly taken care of and would go over every day to check on her and see how she was doing.

One night the neighbour came over and asked me for help. Their cat had gone into labour and something was wrong. When I arrived and felt her belly, I knew in my heart that the cat was in trouble and needed to have a cesarean section immediately. The husband gave me an odd look but took the cat to the vet. After they returned he wanted to know how I had known that the cat needed surgery but I was afraid to tell him. They were very grateful for my help even though they had lost all the kittens. The mother had survived; that was all that mattered to them.

After it was all over I remember sitting in my room and looking at my hands, wondering how I knew what to do and that's when I realized that when I touched people I knew things. I felt scared and sad at the same time because I didn't know what to do with this knowledge. Something shut down inside me then. It was like I had closed a door somewhere inside of myself. Shortly afterwards, I began to suffer debilitating migraines.

As a result of the migraines, the next thirty years became an endless journey of doctors, allopathic medicine, alternative health care, herbs and psychics. Nothing seemed to alleviate the problem and I became increasingly frustrated. Years passed.

One night, in my forties, I had a dream. I dreamt that there was a huge boil on my face. I stood and looked at it in the mirror and as I did, it grew bigger and bigger. I took a needle from the drawer and pierced it. As I squeezed it a huge, pearl white scarab came out of my face. At that point I sat up in sheer terror. I found the dream very disturbing but it was a year and half later that I realized what the dream meant. When I discovered that it meant a spiritual awakening I decided to review my journals and realized that the beginning of my awakening had actually started to unfold ten years earlier.

When I was 32, I suffered a cluster syndrome of migraines that left me almost totally weak on the right side for over six weeks. I started to have dreams about dolphins pulling me into the ocean and meeting a wise Chinese man with five animals made of porcelain at his feet. I had dreams of going through doors and not wanting to look back and dreams where I was handed objects that foretold my future. All of these dreams were very confusing for me because at that time I didn't really dream that much and if I did, rarely remembered them.

In 1995, I began the final journey that would bring me to my knees and almost to the point of death. When I turned 40, my family and I decided to move to Guelph, Ontario. I had returned to school at the time and came home one day to find my husband reading a newspaper.

"Bert, I said, we have to move."

"I know," he replied.

The urge to move came out of nowhere; we were in not in a strong financial situation to make a move but intuitively I knew we had to go. Within a month we were living in Guelph. Shortly afterwards I began to get increasingly ill from the migraines. They were escalating in intensity and it was taking longer to recover from each episode. I started to develop other physical symptoms such as dramatic weight loss, constipation and anemia. This was also when I remembered a vision that I had as a child that told me I would die in my 45th year. It didn't scare me; I just accepted it as fact. Unbeknownst to my family, I was secretly making funeral arrangements including picking out hymns and deciding where I wanted my ashes scattered.

Even though I had accepted my death, I began to work with a doctor again in order to cope with my remaining years. I kept telling my doctor, "There's something wrong here. It's not just migraines, there's something more going on with my body." My doctor just laughed and told me "it was all in my head" and for the next five years we were locked in a very tense battle of wills. The doctor tried very hard to get me on antidepressant medication and into therapy because she thought my physical symptoms were psychosomatic. Even though she was the expert, I trusted my intuition that said that there was something else very, very wrong and that I was running out of time. I knew I had to take action.

In 1999 I began to collapse at work. The doctors told me I was suffering from anxiety and suggested that I take time off. I knew it wasn't anxiety but I was becoming weaker daily and no longer had the will to fight anyone. I took to my bed. After a month of sleeping almost 23 hours a day I realized that I could no longer stand up and walk. I would have to roll myself out of bed and crawl on my hands and knees to the bathroom. My family was pretty self-sufficient by this time so I was not needed around the house, which was a blessing in disguise. I began to notice that there seemed to be a funny odour in the bedroom that was vaguely familiar but I couldn't quite place it.

One afternoon I awoke to find an angel standing beside my bed. She smiled at me and said: "It is your choice, you can live or you can die." At first I thought I was having a hallucination but then I realized what she was saying was the truth. I had to decide. That's when I realized that the odour I couldn't identify in my room was the smell of my own death. I had just turned 45 a few days earlier. It dawned on me that I didn't have much more time.

At first I said, "Take me, I can't do this anymore. I give up." I became aware of floating upwards and I was filled with such heavenly peace. Then I stopped. I thought about my husband and my children and realized that I couldn't leave them alone like that. I called out to the angels and said, "Can I change my mind, please? I would like to choose life." I felt someone smile and heard "Yes." I fell into a deep sleep. When I woke up the next day I felt a lot better. I was able to get up, eat and actually sit up for a little while, something I had not been able to do for over a month.

Russ Mater was a cranial sacral therapist that I had been seeing for my migraines, and had really been helping me get through the previous three months. He suggested I see a practitioner by the name of Larry Steel who did energy work. I had no desire, nor the energy to drive the four hours to see someone who did something I didn't know anything about. Every time I saw Russ he would tell me to see Larry and I would refuse to go. Now I realized that I had to go. I called Larry's office and got an appointment to see him in two weeks.

In the meantime, my boss phoned my doctor because he was concerned for my wellbeing and didn't feel I was getting the help that I needed. He insisted that the doctor do additional tests and this is when I was told that maybe I had celiac disease (CD), a medical condition in which the absorptive surface of the small intestine is damaged by a substance called gluten. Basically, it is a severe food allergy to wheat, rye, spelt, oats, kamut and barley. As a former registered medical technologist I had been trained to believe that CD was always diagnosed in the first four years of life due to failure to thrive. Although I did not feel that I had this problem, I was impressed that she was actually willing to investigate further because up to this time, she had flatly refused. A few days later I went for an upper gastrointestinal X-ray series. The radiologist in charge of the lab came up to me after the tests and asked me what the problem was. I told him my symptoms and the struggle I had been having with my doctor. He asked me if I would be willing to stay for another hour and do some additional tests. He couldn't understand how things had gone on this long and was concerned about my physical condition.

By this time I had dropped down to a weight of 98 lbs and had difficulty standing. I was passing out in the waiting room while I waited for the test results. Finally, the radiologist came to me and said he needed to show me something. He took me into his office and up on the wall were all the X-rays of my abdomen. There was a very large white mass that ran from one side to the other. I got very calm.

"It's not cancer," he said.

"I know," I said.

"Something is very wrong here and you need to have a biopsy. You will have to get your doctor to order a biopsy."

"That will never happen," I said. "I have been fighting with her for five years and she has always refused to run additional tests in the past."

He hesitated because he said doctors couldn't tell each other what to do. I told him that I had worked in hospitals long enough to know that there were always ways around that.

"You have to help me," I said. If you can't be an advocate for me, I'm dead."

He did.

The next day I got a call from my doctor's office asking me to come in right away. I was booked for a biopsy a week later.

In the meantime I knew time was running out and I wasn't sure I was going to make it to my biopsy or to the appointment to see this energy healer, Larry Steel.

The day before the appointment to see Larry I was worried that my husband wasn't going to be able to drive me. I could only sit up for five minutes at a time and driving for four hours was out of the question. My husband assured me that he would take me and if he couldn't (he worked on call seven days a week) that he had made arrangements with a neighbor to take me. On the morning of my appointment, my husband was called in to work at five a.m. He told me not to worry and called the neighbor but they couldn't take me either because the whole family had been up all night with the flu. I thought, "The flu in July?" I just looked at my husband and said, "OK, I will drive myself. I have to go."

I got into the car and started to drive down the highway. After about 20 minutes of driving I was shaking with fatigue and could barely keep the car on the road. I started to cry and looked up at heaven and said: "God, if you want me there that badly, then you are going to have to make this happen, because I am turning this car around and going back home." The next thing I knew, four hours later, I was pulling into Larry's parking lot. I had never been there before; how could I possibly have gotten there? I don't know how but I was relieved to have made it.

I will never forget my first impressions of Larry Steel. I came into his office and sat in the hallway overlooking his treatment room. Here was a young man who looked to be about 16 years old, waving his hands over a woman lying down on a table. I just sat there in stunned silence and said to myself: "God, surely you are crazy. This can't possibly help." All I heard in response was "Wait".

A short time later the front door opened and a man and an older woman carried a middle-aged woman into the office. They laid her down in front of me and started to unwrap her leg, which was totally black. I was shocked. I looked at her leg and said, "Shouldn't you be in a hospital?" She just smiled and said she had just been discharged. It turned out she was American and the doctors couldn't figure out what had happened to her leg and wanted to amputate. The problem for her and her elderly mother was the fact that they would both have to sell their homes to pay for the surgery. She would lose her job and the family would be forced onto welfare. This is the cost of health care to families in the United States. She told me she had heard about Larry and decided that she had nothing to lose except her leg, which could happen anyway. I just shrugged my shoulders and thought "Good luck!"

Now it was my turn to see Larry. He didn't say a word. He just looked at my chart and asked me what my primary concern was.

"I get really bad migraines," I told him.

"OK," was all he said.

I lay down on the table and the minute he touched me I could feel my energy shift. After two minutes he said, "OK, you're done."

I sat up and asked, "What's wrong with me?"

"You have celiac disease," he said.

I was stunned. I had not told him what the doctors suspected. I had never even told him that I was going in for a biopsy. I asked him, "Now what?"

"Come back in an hour and we will work on you some more," he said.

I received five treatments that day. When I drove home that night I cried all the way home. When I walked through the door my husband looked at me and said, "What happened? You look great."

"I think I have been healed," I said.

He thought that was preposterous but said, "Well you look great so if it is working, great."

Two days later my biopsy confirmed celiac disease. The doctor who performed the biopsy said it was the worst case of CD he had ever seen and it was a miracle I was still alive. I just smiled.

For the next three months I returned to Larry's office and would stay for two days receiving five treatments each day. Whenever I returned to Larry's office I would run into the American woman with the black leg. Over the next three months I was a witness to her leg going from black to green to blue to baby pink. Within three months she had fully recovered and had full use of her leg. It was a miracle. Little did I know that God was providing me with visual proof that there was something to this energy work.

During my sessions with Larry I didn't say much. He would occasionally ask me a question or two but for the most part, it was healing as usual. One day he looked down at me and said, "What do you do for a living?" I told him I was a manager at a crop insurance company.

"Are you happy there?" he asked.

"Yes," I replied.

"You could do healing work too you know," he said.

"What, are you nuts?"

He just smiled and told me to think about it. "When you are ready to begin your training, let me know," he said.

I just shook my head. When I told my husband what he had said later that day, Bert replied, "What, is he nuts?"

I thought about it for two months and then thought: "Why not? I don't have anything to lose." I called him up and said, "OK, I'll do the training."

"Great," he said. "But first you have to train with Lori Wilson and take her channeling course."

I'd never heard of channeling but thought OK, if that is what I need to do, I'll do it.

When I showed up at Lori's class I knew I was in for something life changing. Despite the fact that my intuition was telling me that this was going to change my life forever, I was really nervous and afraid that I had absolutely no business playing around with this stuff. When I sat down with the other women in the group I felt very intimidated. They were all experienced in healing work in one way or another. There was a chiropractor, some Reiki Masters, a naturopath, massage therapists, some social workers and me, "Little Miss Corporate". I felt way out of my element. I took a deep breath and plunged in.

The very first exercise that she took us through was teaching us to connect to our higher self. Within the first five minutes, I got it. I was flying. When I "saw" my higher self I said, "Yea, yea, I know you all ready; where is he, where is he?" And then I saw HIM. I looked at my guide and burst into tears. This was the voice, the guide, the one person I had been able to count on since my earliest childhood memories.

"Who are you?" I asked.

When he started to say his name I finished it for him. It was Master Chui Lai. I called him "Grandfather."

After the exercise Lori came up to me and very lovingly said, "Atherton, you don't need to be here anymore. You have found everything you need to find."

"No, I am staying, I want to know everything." Even though I knew she was right. I had found what I was looking for; I just didn't want to miss anything she had to teach. But in reality I spent the next three days just talking to Grandfather when we did any of the other exercises to explore different sources of wisdom.

A short time later, I woke up one night to find the bedroom filled with every kind of door imaginable; doors of every shape, size, and colour. At first I was confused and stood amazed as every door slammed open and fell away. I heard, "Bang, bang, bang" and then they were all gone and there was nothing but openness. After it was over I understood that the pathway for me was now totally open. I was told that all the obstacles were now removed and I could train to be an energy healer.

I recalled Christ's command to acknowledge and accept this gift. Jesus says: *"Truly, truly, I say to you. He who believes in me will also do the works that I do; and greater works than these will he do, because I go to the Father. Whatever you ask in my name, I will do it, that the Father may be glorified in the Son; if you ask anything in my name, I will do it."* *John 14 v 12-14*[16]

In November of that year I began my training as an energy healer with Larry Steel. It took a year to receive my certification. As soon as I did, I left my corporate job, opened my own office and had a full time practice within three months. Over the next three years I continued training in numerous healing modalities to further hone my intuitive abilities. I have never looked back and see each day as a miracle and am honoured to be doing this work.

When that final moment of awareness that I was a healer became evident to me, it flowed quietly into my consciousness like a gentle

---

[16] Harper Study Bible. Revised Standard Version 1962.

stream. As I stood there, in the middle of this stream, there was clarity; an understanding of every decision, all the tears I'd shed, moments of anger, frustration and all the decisions I had made in the past were an important part of the final outcome. I just knew and it felt so very right.

Years later I realized that my vision of dying in my 45th year was not about my physical death, but my spiritual death. They call this experience the *shaman's death*. From that moment on, I was reborn. My life came into focus and began to truly flow.

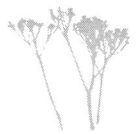

THE SCARAB
THE GIFT OF POWER SYMBOLS

As I mentioned in an earlier chapter, I had a dream ten years ago that was deeply significant to my awakening as a healer. In the dream, I woke up one morning to find a very large sore on my right cheek. Instinctively I knew that I needed to open the sore up and drain it. When I did that, a large mother of pearl scarab slipped out of the sore. It shocked me so much that I woke up suddenly with a gasp. The dream really shook me up and I spent the next year and half thinking about it every day, wondering what it meant. I asked a lot of people for their opinion but they all said the same thing: "What does it mean to you?" It was very frustrating because I was hoping that they could tell me the significance of the dream.

A year and half later we decided to drive into Toronto with the children to see the Egyptian artifact display at the Royal Ontario Museum. As we were walking around we came to a display that showed a model pyramid. At the base of one of the pyramids were little carved scarabs. In front of one of the scarabs was a placard that read: *Scarabs were given to initiates to signify their awakening to the mystic journey*. I was stunned and suddenly understood the significance of the dream.

My mother had spent my whole life training me to open up to my spiritual abilities and I was never sure if what she was teaching me was having an effect. I knew that I was intuitive and it often made other people around me uncomfortable so I spent most of my life hiding it. Only my mother and my husband were aware of the transitions that I was going through. There were many times I felt that pursuing my spiritual awareness created more problems in my life. And yet there was this unusual synchronicity at major turning points that kept me on the path of enhancing my spiritual awareness and understanding how to use my intuitive abilities. I realized in that moment, looking at the scarab in the museum, that the dream was a sign from my angel guides that I was on the right path.

The scarab then became a concrete symbol for me that what I was doing was right. When you're consciously working with angels and guides they will find ways to answer you with concrete symbols. If I go to my angel guides to ask for proof, "Is this the right thing to do for me?" and I see my symbol, I know they are answering my question in the affirmative. To this day the scarab remains a very powerful symbol in my life and in my work.

Symbols will often act as a signpost that a transition or dramatic change is about to take place in your life or confirm the right decision has been made. The truth of this symbol played out in a dramatic way during a very turbulent time in my life.

Larry Steel was the first person to show me that my gifts of intuition could be of service to others. A year after I finished my training with him, I had already begun to develop a full time practice doing healing work out of my home. One day as I sat in meditation I was given a vision of a house where I was told I would move my practice. I made a note of the vision and thought nothing of it again for five years.

Then one day, Archangel Michael and Archangel Gabriel came to me and told me it was time to move my practice out of the house. I spent the next year and half looking for a building to help fulfill this vision. But every door seemed closed to me. I didn't realize until later that I was being educated by the angels on everything I needed to know to make the business a reality including by-laws, zoning, pricing, taxes, and licenses. There were numerous times I would go back to the angels in frustration and say: "OK guys, not getting this. You said it was time to move but I am not getting a whole lot of encouragement or support here." They would just stand there and smile at me. I knew that meant I just had to have faith and keep looking because when the timing was right it would all fall into place.

One day I ran into a friend who knew of my vision and he asked me if I had found the house yet. I just sighed and said, "I give up. I have had enough. No more looking or trying!" Five minutes later, literally, as I drove up a street, I saw a "For Sale" sign and heard Archangel Michael say to me: *"That's the house."*

I immediately slammed on my brakes, and quickly whipped the car around the corner – it is only by the grace of God that the woman behind me didn't smack into the back of my car. I parked the car, pulled out my cell phone and called my real estate agent.

James Nagy is a very busy guy and is never in his office. Imagine my surprise when he picked up the phone. I told him that I wanted to see the house and he got me an appointment. Later that night, when my husband and I walked into the house, I knew this was it. Even our agent, who always thought me sweet but a little kooky (he calls me an "earth muffin") just smiled and said, "Yep, this is the place for you." Two hours later, our offer was accepted.

The next day, when the financial reality dawned on us, we began to panic. To calm myself down, I felt that I needed to walk through the house by myself with my angel guides to reassure me. The owner was very generous and gave me permission to take all the time I needed. As I walked around upstairs I suddenly had a funny feeling. I stopped and turned around to find the spirit of my mother standing in the room with me. She smiled and said, "Do you want the house?"

I said, "Yes, very much."

"Then it is yours," she said and disappeared.

Then I called in the Archangel Michael and asked him if I was really supposed to go through with this. "If this is really the house," I said to him, "then I need tangible proof from you. I need something in my hands that I can hold onto. Give me something that I can hold and keep so that I know without a doubt that this house and that vision is the truth and we are being guided through this."

Archangel Michael smiled and disappeared.

"It drives me crazy when he does that," I said to myself but I did feel calmer and proceeded to walk into the next room. When I entered that room, I heard his voice.

"Look in the corner," he said.

I turned and in the corner, on the floor was a jeweled scarab pin. That's when I knew that this was the right house and that everything would fall into place. And it did.

Every day is an honour and a blessing to be here at the Paradigm Centre for Wellness. My colleagues and I have been able to help so many people on their healing journey. Every day we have clients that remark on what a beautiful, loving space this is. Every client also says the same thing. "When you enter the house you feel loved, safe and know that you have come to the right place."

We all smile, knowing this house is a gift from the angels. That scarab is proof that the vision they gave me would become reality. To this day that scarab is framed and in a special place in my treatment room.

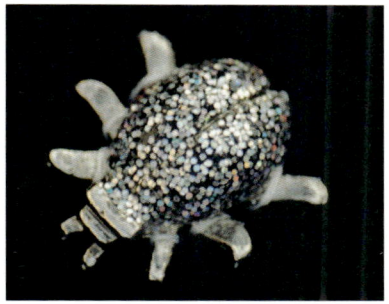

How To Receive Your Power Symbol

Everyone can be gifted a symbol that will be their confirmation that their guides are working with them. If you would like to find out what your symbol is, when you go to bed at night, ask that you be shown in your dreams what your personal symbol is and that you will remember it when you wake up. The next day, allow yourself to be aware of what is presented to you and don't doubt it. If you find that you doubt the symbol, that's just your ego mind getting in the way. You will know soon enough that the symbol is true for you.

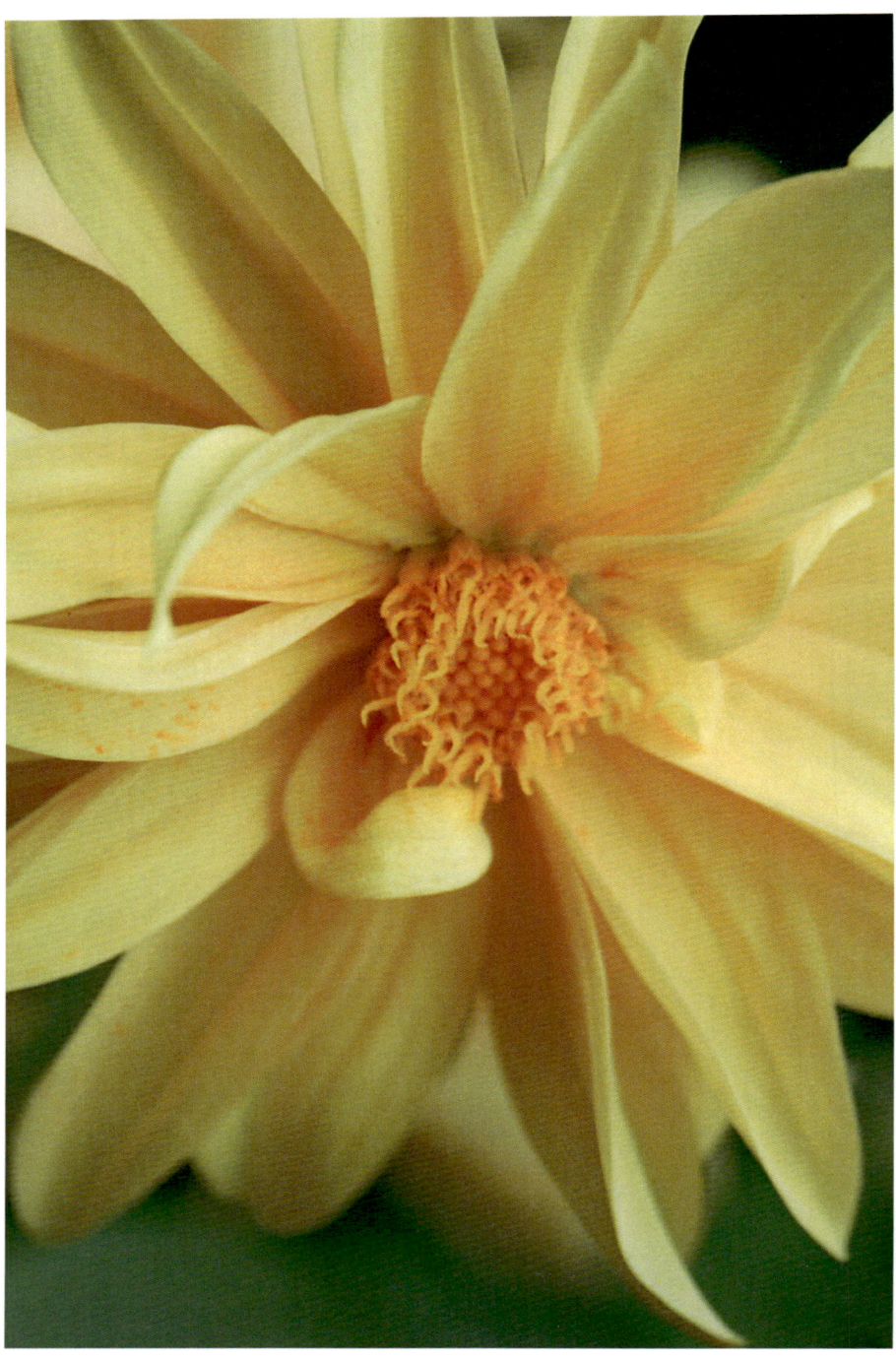

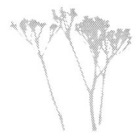

Case Histories

In the following chapters you are going to read the stories of some of my clients who chose to try healing using energy medicine. It is a privilege to share their stories so that others can understand the power of this work and how it can be of service to them.

The following stories have been published with permission but names and identifying details have been changed to protect each family's identity.

EMBEDDED MEMORIES

To better understand the following case histories, we need to understand how energy medicine releases embedded memories. For example, do you find that even though you have spent time in therapy to resolve a memory or issue it continues to resurface and have an impact on your life? Would you be amazed to learn that your memories will always be there? Would you be startled to learn that the feelings that go with those memories will also always be there? Clients often say for every two steps that they take forward they feel that they are taking one step backwards. Discouraging isn't it?

There are two ways of handling a memory. One, you can recoil from the pain and shock the memory creates and try to bury it again in the subconscious, the results of which can cause anxiety or create any other form of emotional turmoil. This type of reaction can sometimes lead to physical symptoms like anxiety, depression, headaches, gut aches and even joint pain. This is because suppressed memories or fear create blockages in the energy field. Or two, you can turn towards the memory and face what has happened and ask yourself, "What did I need to learn here?" This second option is called *coming into conscious awakening*. This can be difficult to do alone and is where a holistic energy therapist can be of assistance.

When we are dealing with memories held within the body, the thing to remember is that energy and memories have no sense of time. A trauma that occurred at birth can still be "present" in a person's energy field. This can create a blockage in the energy field that acts like a small grain of sand. Each passing day or each passing experience begins to coat the little grain of sand until it becomes like a stone. The stone can then grow, with further life experience, becoming bigger and bigger until it resembles a boulder.

In energy work when you uncover an old memory, your body wisdom is giving you an opportunity to review your belief system at the moment when the memory occurred and bring it to light so that you can see it in a different way. This *conscious awakening* empowers you because you're put in a position to reevaluate what you experienced and how you translated that experience into a belief system. This shifts your emotional reaction and helps you to understand what you were trying to learn. In effect it changes your reaction to this past traumatic event, restructures your view of current events and impacts future events. It also gives the body permission to release and heal old wounds held in the energy field because the emotional trauma is no longer seen as a threat. This is called a *healing miracle*.

When you are in session and the memory resurfaces, you are guided into observing the memory by the HET, as if you were watching a movie. And this is a key point. You are only remembering the story, not reliving the incident and recalling the judgements that you made in that moment. The healer helps you to safely observe the different emotions that occurred at that time and uncover the core beliefs that were created.

The healer helps to hold you safe while you remember. This allows you to be the calm observer of the past. As you replay the memory you have the opportunity to acknowledge and name the feelings that occurred. Then in the midst of the memory the healer will ask you: "What were you looking to learn from this?" The healer is guiding you to safely face your past and acknowledge your emotions and fears.

The way this is done in a session is as follows: The body will indicate that there is a blockage; the healer will go into the blockage and find out what statement of belief is being held there; at what age it became imprinted; and then the healer voices it back to the client.

The healer will then ask the client what they remember happening at that age. The client always goes right to the story, even if they say they have no memory of their childhood. The client will then describe the memory and the healer will ask them what were they looking to learn. The client often realizes in a moment what occurred and why they decided on that belief. When that happens the body will release the blockage and the energy field or aura will begin to flow again around that area. Clients will experience a sensation of relief; they will sigh, they may cry, they can laugh and their body will just physically relax on the table.

In one case, blockage is discovered around the gall bladder. The statement is – *seething resentment.* The healer will ask "Age?" and the body responds, *"Age eight"*. The healer then asks the client: "What happened at age eight that made you feel seething resentment?" The client remembers that her parents promised to buy her a pony if she was a good girl all year. She struggled all year in school to get good marks, which resulted in constant gut aches. When it came time to buy the pony her parents just laughed and told her not to be ridiculous – they never had any intention of buying her a pony. She decided that *people that you love, always lie to you*. Not only did she suffer from constant gallbladder attacks as a young adult, she couldn't stay in a relationship long enough to get married.

People can be afraid of a memory because they've built it up so much in their minds that they think there is something horrible in the memory that can never be healed. It looms like a dark cloud over their head. This is why they eventually come to see a healer – they can't bear to live with this cloud obstructing the joy and love in their lives.

The following case history further illustrates the impact of embedded memories and how they were released through the process of energy work.

Additional case histories follow to illustrate how energy medicine can help heal.

JUDY
RELEASING EMBEDDED MEMORIES

A young mother, by the name of Judy came to the Centre suffering from constant anxiety. Judy said that the anxiety had become so intense that she was finding it harder to care for her young family as well as herself. Judy rarely left the house except to walk her children to school and to go grocery shopping. Judy had tried therapy and anti-depressants but nothing helped; her condition continued to get worse.

In the first session, when we went to body wisdom to find the root cause of her anxiety, body moved me into the emotional field of her aura and here we found a blockage over the solar plexus that had been present from the age of 18 months. I asked Judy what had happened in her life when she was 18 months old. She remembered that was when her baby brother had been born. She was surprised to remember how upset she had been with her parents for having another baby. She thought that she was their baby and couldn't understand why she didn't matter anymore to her parents. As a result of this Judy realized she had become afraid that her parents were going to leave her somewhere because they didn't need her anymore. After all, the small child in her reasoned, they got a new toaster when the old one didn't work anymore. She thought she would be replaced in the same way. Her young child mind believed that she was replaceable. This was the seed of the fear in her.

Shortly thereafter, Judy began to develop all sorts of "little fears." Her family found her fears amusing and would tease her about them at family gatherings. This made the fears worse and Judy began to develop fears about going to family gatherings and would often develop headaches to avoid them. As she got older she was became more and more reclusive. By the time Judy was a mother her fearfulness was so intense she could barely step outside the house.

Over the next several months we worked in her emotional field with the anxiety and her fears. We often returned to this painful event of her parents bringing her brother home from the hospital. Eventually Judy was able to walk back into the memory of seeing her brother for the first time. As she watched the movie in her mind's eye Judy allowed herself to feel the fear. As she experienced the fear she recognized that she felt she was being pushed aside. It made her feel sad and abandoned. She began to understand the story. Here was a small child, who until her brother showed up felt all of her parents' love and devotion. But the small child felt that her parents' attention to the baby meant that they didn't love her anymore. This made her sad. She was too young to understand how to cope with this new emotion of sadness; sadness developed into fear. As time went on, and her brother grew older Judy would feel sad every time her parents paid attention to her brother. This created more fear.

Eventually the fears were connected to various events. Because the events were physical and her parents could see and react to the physical, the fears would become embedded in the event. If she and her brother were playing and her brother cried, Judy would be blamed for "hurting the baby". Therefore Judy became afraid of hurting others and felt compelled to watch and monitor everything she said and did. As a result of the embedded memory, Judy became shy and socially awkward. Talking to strangers was almost agonizing.

If Judy and her brother were out playing a game and her brother won, her parents would praise her brother for winning. Judy embedded this memory as evidence that her brother was better than her. Judy grew up believing that her brother was always better than she was at anything. Judy never did really well at school because she thought she wasn't as good. She chose to go to work after high school instead of going to university. She couldn't bear the thought of having to compete with her brother.

When Judy came home from school with her report card her parents would comment on how well she was doing. When her brother showed his report card they would also comment on how well he was doing but Judy didn't see that. She only saw that his marks were better than hers. Judy felt that they should look at her report card and comment on the lower marks and then realize that she was struggling and try to help her. But instead, in their efforts to be fair and loving to her, they would just praise her efforts. This was not being honest, as far as Judy was concerned. This memory reinforced Judy's belief that "people are not honest and can't be trusted". This created more fear in her.

When the adult mind understood the root cause of the fear, she realized that she had nothing to truly fear. Judy's parents loved her and they just happened to have had another baby. When Judy faced this memory and all of its emotions, she suddenly understood that her fears were of her own making. She had never understood her own fear of abandonment but now as an adult she totally understood how it contributed to all these "little fears". Judy was now able to embrace this memory. As she wiped away her tears she laughed at how scared she'd been for all of those years and she felt free for the first time in her adult life. Judy now felt she was open to really seeing her brother as a friend and not a threat to her anymore.

Over the next several sessions, all these fears began to untangle themselves from her memories. She could look on each memory with a fresh perspective. She could look at each memory and "see" where she felt sad and rejected. Judy chose to understand what was really happening with each memory. Each story was about a little girl who felt sad because of her belief. She realized that the belief was not the truth. The truth was that her parents loved and cherished her and they did the same for her brother. "That awareness changed everything for me," Judy said.

The next time Judy feels abandonment, she will understand where that fear is coming from. She will acknowledge it and realize that she no longer needs to be manipulated by that belief system. The memory is there, but the pain is gone and there is love and understanding with what she remembers now. With this realization comes *conscious awareness*.

As a result of this, Judy now understands that she is not taking two steps forward and one step back. Remembering is not going backwards in this process; it is moving forward with conscious awareness and exercising choice.

After extensive work over several months, Judy is now actively involved in her community and her children's school. She is considering applying to university part time to obtain her degree – a dream she has always had. This story is a good example of how energy work transforms fear.

Basically there are only two emotions – love and fear. The goal of energy work is to transform fear into love. Only by addressing the fear can this process begin.

How Did Energy Work Help Judy?

Judy suffered from constant anxiety that resulted in her being unable to leave her home and care for her young family.

Energy work helped Judy to identify that the root cause for her anxiety stemmed from a childhood memory of believing that she was being rejected by her parents when her brother was born. As a young child, Judy felt deep sadness and was unable to cope with the emotion. Her consciousness dealt with the sadness by turning it into fear; her parents gave her attention when she was fearful.

Once Judy understood the root cause of her fear, she made conscious decisions around what she was truly feeling and chose to change her belief systems. As a result of her *conscious awakening* around her fears, and changing her beliefs, Judy was able to overcome these fears and live an active, productive life.

KATRINA
RELEASING FEAR AND LEARNING HOW TO LIVE IN GRATITUDE

Katrina came to the practice to see if she could be helped with her overwhelming fears for her grandson. She also realized that she had self -esteem issues that were unresolved and felt that she was a "people pleaser" and never felt good enough. When she was younger she had suffered from an eating disorder but after years of therapy this was now resolved. Twelve years ago she was diagnosed as Type I diabetic. The onset of this disease came without warning, she told me. One day she was fine, the next she was diagnosed with diabetes.

Katrina was born in a small country in eastern Europe. Both of her parents were born during World War II. When she was two years old her parents got divorced; she never saw her birth father again. When she was five years old her mother remarried. A short time after her mother remarried, the Communists came to power. Her mother and stepfather decided they needed to escape the country and had to leave Katrina behind with her mother's parents. It took her mother five years to get her out. While she remained behind she lived with her grandparents, whom she adored. She was able to keep in touch with her mother through cassette tapes. She was happy and had a wonderful life. One day her grandparents told her that she was leaving for Canada. Katrina was put on a plane, by herself and sent to Canada. She was ten years old, terrified and devastated to be taken away from her grandparents. When she arrived in Canada and met her mother for the first time in five years, her mother had a baby girl in her arms. Katrina hadn't been told that she had a sister; it was all very confusing for her. Her first year in Canada was a blur. She was put in a school and didn't know how to speak English or understand it. No one helped her, not even her parents. When she complained and said she wanted to go home, her mother would tell her that she lived in Canada now and needed to get used to it. But no one explained to her what that meant or how to do it. "I don't think my parents understood the trouble I was having assimilating into a new culture," she said. "I felt it was 'sink or swim for me.' I never received any emotional support."

Katrina hated her new little sister and felt that her sister got everything she needed and yet Katrina was left to suffer it out alone. She had a lot of resentment towards her sister and her mom.

When Katrina was twelve years old she was molested by a pedophile. Because she was so desperate for attention it happened more than once. She didn't realize that it was wrong until it was too late. Again, knowing that she couldn't talk to her mother about anything emotional, she suffered in silence and developed bulimia a short time later. By this age she realized how fearful her mother was. Having grown up during the war and then suffering through the aftermath had left her mother emotionally scarred, frightened and closed down.

Katrina was very young when she married for the first time. She just wanted to get out and have a life of her own. They had a son a short time later. After he was born Katrina realized that her husband had a drinking problem. She left him and has never been in contact with him since. She raised her son on her own and a few years later met the love of her life. Her current marriage is strong and her husband supportive. It was with his help that she was able to go into therapy and deal with a lot of her past issues and finally resolve her issues with bulimia.

At Katrina's first session, after we had finished reviewing her life history we went to the body and asked it to "show path to helping her resolve her fears." I immediately could "perceive" cords that came into her body around the abdomen and involved the liver, spleen, pancreas and stomach. These energetic cords are called *fear cords*[17] and they had originated from her grandparents and her birth dad. Fear cords are energetic cords that are very common between parents and their children. They develop when a parent is afraid that if the child doesn't do what they were told to do and gets hurt, the parent will feel that, "It's all my fault." The parent's fear will create a cord that will carry a belief pattern on it. In this instance the fear cord could carry the belief pattern: "If you are not careful you will fall down a staircase."

Let's look at a practical example of how a fear cord can be created and what the end result can be. A parent sees her son John playing with his toy car at the top of a staircase. The mother says, "John if you don't move you could fall down the staircase." John continues to play with his toy car, oblivious to the danger that his mother can see as a possible outcome. Seeing that John has decided to ignore her, she becomes fearful. This fear is projected from the mother toward the son, and is energetically sent out as a cord of protection because the mother does not want her son to fall down the staircase.

The son now is faced with two choices, either refusing the fear cord or accepting it. Let's look at each scenario and the possible outcomes.

In the first instance John refuses the fear cord. He decides to ignore his mother and continues to play at the top of the stairs. He knows he is

---

[17] See Glossary

loved, but knows how to be careful and therefore does not accept his Mother's fear of possible outcomes. The fear cord does not go into his field and dissolves when the mother realizes that if he does fall, he has been warned, refused to heed her advice and knows that he will learn from experience that playing at the top of stairs isn't a safe decision.

In the second choice, John decides to listen to his mother and accepts the fear cord into his field, feels her fear, and moves away from the staircase and plays somewhere else as a result. He has learned, as a result of his mother's advice that staircases are dangerous and you cannot play there.

In normal circumstances this happens every day, in every household. Parents loving their children and wanting to keep them safe, offer advice on a regular basis and this helps their children understand the world and helps them to make decisions based on experience and sound reasoning. In this case, the staircase is not a safe place to play.

Fear cords become a problem when there is a lot of anxiety around everything. The cords get tangled and the messages get blurred. It is like having too many crossed wires and the emotional body hits an overload and begins to shut down. This can result in fears and phobias that just don't seem to make any sense or, as one client put it, fear that "comes out of nowhere."

In Katrina's case there were a lot of fear cords in her field but there were three major cords that took on the appearance, weight and texture of tree trunks. They created a lot of energetic drain on her overall field. These fear cords came from three people in her life: her grandparents and her birth father. In each cord there was "war trauma". All three of these people had lived through World War II, in an area where there was a lot of fighting. They had survived food shortages, German occupation, death, destruction, starvation, disease, and the constant fear of never knowing if they were going to live to see another day. Katrina was conceived after the war when the country was trying to rebuild itself. Again during her mother's pregnancy, there were food shortages and constant upheaval. By the time she was five years old her country was being taken over by the Communists.

All three of these fear cords contained the emotional beliefs learned at an energetic level by her grandparents and parents. These belief systems were passed on to her energetically at her conception and were frequently reinforced by her family as she was being raised. These fears where being manifested around her daily as seen in her statement: "My mother was afraid of everything and there was never any emotional support."

After these three fear cords were removed, I went into the body's DNA structure and worked with the body's energy to help it release "war trauma" belief systems learned by her parents and grandparents.

Two weeks later when Katrina contacted me for another session she said, "I have had a phenomenal two weeks. All the fear I had around my grandson is gone. I can finally just enjoy him. What can I do to feel this way all the time about everything in my life?"

> ### *Emotional Trauma and DNA Patterning*
> What I've witnessed through my work is that emotional traumas create belief systems which produce an energetic pattern that gets imprinted onto the DNA. This energetic pattern can be passed on from generation to generation. Energy medicine can often work with this patterning and help to release it.

I said, "Let's see what the body and soul are ready to release and help with the healing." When we worked together in this session, the body's wisdom took us to issues around self-doubt. The body showed us there were beliefs that said, "I'm not worth it" and "self punishment". At this point we were shown that there was a split in the soul path[18] at age 14. And a piece of her was still stuck in that age and needed to be brought forward and reunited with her soul path at her current age to help the body and soul feel whole and complete once again. We then helped the body to adjust to this energetic part that was reunited with her energy field again.

When Katrina called two weeks later, she said that she felt pretty good. "I'm on a roll," she said. You could tell that she was beginning to see what could be resolved and healed using energy medicine and was anxious for more. She had started to take a good hard look at how she was feeling about different things in her day-to-day life. This was perfect because now she was making conscious choices about what she wanted to believe and not believe. She noticed that she was afraid to make

---

[18] See Glossary

choices about anything. She found herself being consumed with fear and realized that being unhappy was more comfortable than being happy, which she found very interesting. She asked, "How do I get out of this?"

When we connected with her body wisdom, about being consumed by fear, the body took us back in time to the abuse with the pedophile. During the periods of abuse it was discovered that she began to believe that she was "incapable or useless." We uncovered fear beliefs that stated "angry with mom for bringing me to Canada", "shock of being taken away from my grandparents" and emotional struggles with "knowing it is OK to be here, in Canada". The clearing of these belief systems wasn't easy. She cried and felt the pain of the fear leaving her. After the session was over she felt lighter and that she had a deeper understanding of why it was so hard for her to feel happy. It had never been safe to be happy after she came to Canada. She realized she had some decisions to make about how she felt daily, based on her life now and not on what she once believed. Katrina was given a homework assignment until her next session. I asked her to answer the question, "What do I need to feel safe?"

At her next session Katrina said her homework helped her to see that she couldn't feel safe until she knew "that I will be OK if something bad happens." For example she said, "I am afraid to buy a new couch because I am afraid that if I buy a new couch and we lose our jobs we can't pay for the couch and then we will be in trouble. So I don't buy the couch until I have all the money saved up. This means we can go for years living with furniture that falls apart and we are miserable." I asked her, "If you believe that you have to know you are safe before you do anything, but believe that you will never be safe, how can you ever feel safe?"

She was puzzled and said, "I don't get it."

I said, "Do you and your husband have good jobs?"

"Yes," she replied.

"Do you and your husband make enough money to live in a home?"

"Yes," she replied.

"Do you make enough money to pay your bills at the end of every month?"

"Yes."

"Do you have money left over at the end of every month?"

"Yes."

"Are you or your husband going to be laid off?"

"No."

"But you live like you are going to lose your jobs tomorrow?"

"Yes, we do."

"Is that the truth?"

"No, it isn't."

"Then why would you live that as your truth?"

"I don't know. I am afraid to be happy. I don't believe I can be happy, therefore I won't buy the couch and the whole family ends up being miserable because of that."

We discussed this further and worked through a couple more examples of what was happening in her daily life that was manifesting her current belief that it wasn't safe to be happy because something bad could happen. She realized that she was standing in her own way of happiness because she "won't let [her] guard down." She goes on to say, "If I do, something bad is bound to happen and it is my way of controlling everything, isn't it?"

"What do you want to do about this?" I asked her.

 "I can't live like this anymore. It is not who I want to be and it is not what I want to teach my children," she said.

Mother Mary stepped forward at this point and said to her:

"Go forward in gratitude, knowing that we are always grateful for you."

We talked about learning how to live in gratitude for what she had and how, despite everything she had been through in life, she had still managed to marry well, be happy, have a great job and money in the bank. I suggested she work with the belief statement: "All my needs are being met on this day."

I suggested that she say this to herself daily, as often as possible, and that she also reinforce this new belief system by daily reminding herself of what she had to be grateful for. I suggested that when returning from work every day she could sit in her driveway and look at her home and feel gratitude. I suggested that she develop a daily practice of letting her husband and children know how grateful she was for them. She could do this by showing gratitude in her eyes when she spoke to them or thanked them for something they had done that day. I suggested that at work each morning she, "Take a few moments to look at the building and give gratitude to your employer and colleagues at work."

How Did Energy Work Help Katrina?

Katrina suffered from overwhelming fears and low self-esteem as a result of her family's belief systems due to their history of war trauma. These emotional beliefs were triggered and reinforced when she immigrated to Canada as young teenager.

Energy work helped Katrina to identify the root cause of her fears and identify her core belief that it was "not safe to be happy because something bad might happen." Katrina was able to change her core belief so that each day she understood all of her needs were being met on that day; consequently, she could practice gratitude for that. Katrina is no longer paralyzed by fear in her life and is able to live joyfully and with gratitude for the abundance that is her life.

SONYA
WORKING WITH FEAR SNAKES

In our work with clients, healers often find fear in one form or another. One of the most interesting types of fear to encounter is in the form of a snake. When fear appears in an energy field in this formation, it usually results from a deeply rooted fear that has been carried since childhood, or has been carried on the soul path[19] as the result of a past life trauma.

Fear snakes can be easy to remove if you are patient and are willing to listen to the story. Fear snakes cannot just be pulled out – they have to be coaxed, often by relaying the story of why they were created in the first place – back to the client. By doing this you are giving the client an opportunity, consciously and subconsciously, to "remember" and then to choose to release the belief that created the fear snake in the first place.

Sonya's story is typical of what happens when a fear snake appears. Fear snakes can be huge and weigh hundreds of pounds energetically or they can be like tiny thread-like worms that just ooze out of the field. In this story I was just beginning to learn how to handle fear snakes, and as is often the case when I encounter something new, I will turn to the angels for instruction and direction.

Sonya is a client that I have never met personally. She lives in another part of the world and we started working together after being

---

[19] See Glossary

introduced over the phone several years ago. When a healer works with a client over the phone like this, it is called *distance work*.[20]

When we do distance work the session has a particular structure. The client calls in at their appointment time. I ask how they have been since our last session and how can I be of service on this day? After the information has been recorded and verbal permission received, I connect to their energy field and bring them in energetically. In my treatment room I have created an energy portal that looks like a lovely white wrought iron gate. Standing on either side of this gate are two angels who call themselves Bill and Bob. When the client is called in energetically they appear at the gate, the angels open the gate, and the client walks in. This portal and these two angels protect the client by allowing only their energy to enter. They also protect me by allowing only the client to enter and making sure the portal is closed, secure and protected during and after a session is over. After the session is completed, the client's energy is escorted back by Archangel Michael to ensure safe journey and protection.

When the client enters the room energetically I watch how they enter and what is happening in their field. (I receive a lot of information about the client in that moment in time.) The images are often very symbolic, as you will see in this case history. Because I have already asked the client how I can be of service before the session begins, her body wisdom is already preparing for the session and choosing where it needs to go for healing.

---

[20] See Glossary

When Sonya appeared energetically in the treatment room she came in wearing a huge snake around her neck. The snake had the appearance of mother of pearl with white, green and blue scales down its back. As this was one of the first times I had dealt with fear snakes of this magnitude, I was unsure of what to do so I turned to the Archangel Michael and asked him for advice.

Archangel Michael said:

"The snake represents her knowledge of how her words can be powerful and dangerous at the same time. We are not to focus on the snake for now but to let her place it to one side."

I relayed this information to Sonya, over the phone, and then energetically we turned away from the fear snake and went to the body energy directly.

I had her lie down on the table energetically and after I had permission from the body wisdom to proceed, the body took us into a protocol I use when dealing with emotional abuse. The body took us back to age eight. At this age Sonya had to appear in court to give testimony against a man who exposed himself to her. It was a frightening time for her and we had been here many times before in previous sessions.

I had Sonya visualize being in the witness box in court giving her testimony. When she was there in memory, the body then allowed us to focus on what it needed to clear at age eight[21]. As we spoke of these

---

[21] When energy blockages are cleared at a certain age, it translates through the energy field to their current age.

things Sonya began to writhe and sob energetically on the table. She said that being on the stand was the most painful thing she had ever done. If she told the court what had happened, this man would be sent to jail. What if he got out? What if he came after her? He attacked her once, what would happen if he did so again? But if she told the truth, other kids would be spared the shame and the horror of what she had been through. If she told her story she knew her parents would be proud of her. At this point, she stopped. She said: "This is the first time I could verbalize what I was feeling on that day. I didn't know the words were in there. I didn't know this is how I really felt. I was just scared all the time. I was always looking for ways to hide myself. If I could make myself ugly, fat or if I could hide somehow (not have people look at me) maybe he couldn't find me again. All I have been doing is hurting myself and punishing my parents because I was afraid." She then started to cry again and said, "Will God forgive me?"

Archangel Michael then said,

"We are not judged by God. We judge ourselves and allow the judgements of others to affect our self-being."

This pearl of wisdom from Archangel Michael opened a whole new vista of understanding for Sonya. She had been struggling with relationships (self, parents, partner, work) all her life. Sonya struggled with obesity and low self-esteem. As a result of this she said, "She felt like a prisoner in her own body".

Sonya smiled and sighed with relief. It finally all made sense to her. With this awareness the fear snake released spontaneously and was received back to heaven by the angels for transformation into love and light for the good of all. Whenever you "remove" something from the body energetically it must be replaced with Christ light[22] to facilitate healing. Her throat chakra opened and expanded; her body sighed with relief.

At Sonya's next session she came in looking lighter and more at peace. She said that she was beginning to understand where all her food phobias were coming from and was feeling confident enough to begin dieting again. But this time in a more healthful manner by choosing the right foods instead of crash dieting.

When we went back to the body, it again asked to return to the story of being eight years old and having to testify in court. This story was being held in the emotional level of her aura and was affecting the physical area of her stomach. When we energetically connected to the physical area of the stomach, I felt that it continued to hold fear and heard the body make the statement "being vulnerable." This meant that the body still held more anger and fear around having to go through the court case and feelings of "not being protected." After this anger and fear were acknowledged, her belly opened up energetically and fear snake energy that looked like little worms came pouring out. We gently removed them and again healed the area with Christ light.

Her body then requested that we return to the memory of the court case once again. When we returned to this image the body went back to the stomach area. This time the story that was being held here was not at age eight but tracked back to age two when her brother was born.

---

[22] Christ light is the way that I refer to the universal healing light. Bringing in healing light is a specific technique that is taught to healers in their training.

This time the emotion being held in the stomach area was hatred. The two year old was furious that her parents had the nerve to have another baby. Before this brother was born she was their world and all attention fell on her. When her brother was born she felt she had been pushed aside. When I relayed this story to Sonya she laughed. She said she could remember always being told, "You have to be quiet; your brother is sleeping." She said, "I never did like him much and we never got along as kids."

After we cleared this emotion the belly again opened up energetically and a creamy white stream of energy started to pour out. This mass felt like liquid marshmallows. It was very sticky and had a slightly acrid smell to it. After it cleared the area was infused with Christ light.

After this balancing Sonya talked about how much she hated authority, especially her parents' authority over her. She related how she spent most of her childhood finding very inappropriate ways to buck their authority.

I asked her how this belief system still served her. She was confused. She knew she hated her parents' authority, but until it was pointed out to her she didn't realize that it was still an issue. Therefore, this belief system of hating authority must still be of service to her in some way. We explored possibilities, each time making sure that she was staying connected to her heart so that she would understand what aspect of the belief was true for her.

In the end we discussed several possibilities, such as, she really needed her parents' love and attention and when she didn't receive it she would feel abandoned. She felt a lot of judgement towards her parents abandoning her for another child (her brother). She also felt anger and abandonment when she was placed in the witness box to testify because her parents had not prepared her for this experience.

We again went back to Archangel Michael's statement:

"We are not judged by God. We judge ourselves and allow the judgements of others to affect our self-being."

This was the other aspect of judgement for her. In this memory, she was holding judgement against her parents because they had another baby. She held judgement against her parents because they didn't protect her the way she felt she needed to be protected when she testified in court. She was holding the energy of anger inside of herself because she couldn't forgive her parents for letting her down.

When she became aware of this, she realized that she needed to forgive her parents for not being who she wanted them to be. Sonya was able at this time to step back from these memories and finally understand how to look at issues with more clarity and without judgement. With this realization her body sighed and all her chakras opened up and released.

At her next session Sonya said she was beginning to lose weight while she was eating normally. This was a first for her.

When we are dealing with memories held within the body, the thing to remember is that energy and memories have no sense of time. A trauma that occurred at birth can still be "present" in a person's energy field.

This can create a blockage in the energy field that acts like a small grain of sand. Each passing day or each passing experience begins to coat the little grain of sand until it becomes like a stone. The stone can then grow, with further life experience, becoming bigger and bigger until it resembles a boulder.

This memory is like a grain of sand embedded in the subconscious, which has no time frame. The ego body[23] begins to use it as a frame of reference. The body tries to deal with the memory in the best way it knows how but, as consciousness in the child grows, so does ego body. The ego body begins to reference all incidents against its own thoughts and beliefs. The memory gets buried deeper and deeper until the end result is a symptom or a feeling that seems to have no known cause. Energy work helps to track back into these blockages to find the grain of sand (fear cord or fear snake). When you find that, the body is most eager to rid itself of the irritant and release it. The physical body is free of interference, and can heal. The emotional body has a new frame of reference or new belief system.

How Did Energy Work Help Sonya?

Sonya struggled with weight problems all of her life, yet she was fed up and knew that dieting was not the answer. She knew that there was a deeper meaning to her weight issues. She was frustrated and unhappy with herself and her life. Sonya turned to energy medicine to see if it could help her find the pieces that were missing.

---

[23] The ego body is created in our consciousness during infancy and is based on our sensory experience of our bodies. It forms the belief that we are distinct from other objects. Energy work helps bring into conscious awareness that the ego body boundary is only a mental construct.

Energy work helped Sonya to identify and remove several major fear snakes and fear cords that created energetic interference in her body located primarily in her digestive system where she had been swallowing her anger, vulnerabilities, and need for attention since childhood.

After these blocks were removed, Sonya found that she could stop the dieting merry-go-round and begin to make healthy choices. She was learning how to love who she was, starting to lose weight naturally and her self-esteem was improving dramatically. Sonya eventually met and married her soul mate and went on to open her own successful business; two dreams she thought were unattainable.

LEA
CHANGING BELIEF SYSTEMS AND DEVELOPING GRATITUDE

Lea and I had been working together for a year on relationship issues both personally and within her family. In the course of the year things had improved dramatically with her children and within her family circle but she was getting very impatient with the process because she still had not found a partner and was tired of being alone.

During her sessions we had been working on belief systems and I had given her several new belief statements (or *mantras*[24]) to work with, which had created positive results on her relationships with her children but had not produced a relationship with a loving partner. When we focused on her goal of finding a relationship we encountered the following beliefs in her emotional and mental fields: "You can never trust a man" and, "Men will always let me down."

She found this to be very curious. After further discussion she admitted to me that every time she went on a date, these two statements were her flags. If she felt or sensed either one of them, there was no second date. The problem with this, for her, is that she went on the date looking for it and as a result, she always found it. I explained to her that just saying the new belief statement wasn't going to be enough if she continued to really hold these beliefs because the Universe was only going to hear what she truly believed and that was "You can never trust a man" and, "Men will always let me down".

---

[24] See Glossary

Naturally she was confused and discouraged. She couldn't understand why just saying the new belief statements didn't create change for her. I explained to her that because she had free will she wasn't allowing herself to change her mind about men and as result she continued to produce her old reality around them. She did not hold the same belief system around her children so she was allowing these relationships to change. When I asked for guidance about her belief system about men, this is what I heard: "Dear God, I want you to work a miracle, but I don't want to have to change my mind about anything." This is a common form of resistance when dealing with internal changes. People think they want to change but there is *subconscious resistance*[25] and fear of what that change will mean to them in their personal lives.

I explained to her that God gave us free will so that we have the freedom to choose whatever we want in our lives. This also means that we have the freedom to choose what we believe about our lives, our world, and ourselves.

God created the law of "Cause and Effect". This means that whatever we believe, that is all that the Universe can create for us. This law honours free will and it does not interfere with choice. And remember God is Love and He does not judge us. We only judge ourselves or are willing to accept the judgement of others.

In meditation, an angel told me once: "Life does not happen to you — you create the experience." I shared this wisdom with Lea because I felt she needed to know that she had the power to create the changes in

---

[25] Also called unconscious fear; see Glossary for additional information

her life that she was seeking even though she didn't realize it at the time. Energy work could help her initiate this process but ultimately the power to create the changes she was looking for was in her hands. I explained to Lea that we needed to find out why she believed what she did. Setting the intent to find the root cause of "You can never trust a man" in her body revealed that at around age six her father had lost his job. He was out of work for over a year and her mother would always say to her, "You can never trust a man". When she remembered this, she understood that it wasn't her truth but her mother's belief, and she was playing it out in her own life. She began to understand that this belief was shaping her reality and was the reason she continued to attract men who couldn't keep a job and always depended on her for a living.

We then asked the body to clarify the root cause of the belief: "Men will always let me down." This belief system stemmed from age 16 when she became ashamed of her father because she realized he had a drinking problem. She wanted her father to be like the other dads who held down jobs and came home every night and played with their children. In her lifetime of partnerships she was diligent about never being involved with men who had drinking problems but they always did something or had characteristics that made her feel "shame" about them. Because these two belief systems were so deeply entrenched and had played out so poignantly in her life, we needed to work with clearing the negative belief systems from her subconscious mind. We did this by choosing belief systems that were positive and clarified what she wanted in a partner. We then had her repeat these positive statements while doing cross-crawl[26] with her eyes open and again with her eyes

---

[26] Brain gym exercise

closed. This is a Brain Gym®[27] exercise that helps to incorporate change into the subconscious mind.

One year later Lea introduced me to her new partner, a lovely man who held a steady job. She was very proud of how he was helping her fix up her home and raise her two children. He was a positive role model and a compassionate helpmate.

Brain Gym®

Brain Gym® is a program of physical movements that enhance learning and performance in all areas. It develops the brain's neural pathways the way nature does – through movement. It helps to reconnect or rebalance the neural network between right and left-brain. This creates improvement with coordination, balance, speech, memory, concentration and can even balance the emotional field. Brain Gym® was developed in the 1970s by educators Dr. Paul Dennison and Gail E. Dennison. For more information go to www.braingym.org

---

HOW DID ENERGY WORK HELP LEA?

Lea wanted to have a loving relationship yet everything she did seemed to end in unhealthy relationships. She was at a loss as to what to do and turned to energy work to see if it would help her.

Energy work helped Lea uncover her old core beliefs of "you can never trust a man" and "men will always let me down". Working with these

---

[27] See textbox

two old beliefs we were able to go back into her childhood memories and find out what created these beliefs. Once she "remembered" the old stories, she was able to unlock her subconscious belief patterns.

> ### *Affirmations*
>
> Affirmations are very powerful but people need to stay focused on a positive frame of mind to overcome the obstacles in their way to the new belief. Obstacles are the universe's way of helping you to clear a lot of past negative beliefs in a hurry. I call them blips.
>
> Emotional thoughts create form which can manifest as obstacles in daily life. Old beliefs have created a concrete reality and now you are living the truth of that reality. The only way that reality can change, is if it is challenged and the obstacle is removed. If you stay firm in your new belief, and trust the outcome, the universe will clear the old obstacle very quickly (blip). The trick is not to panic and give up on the new belief. Stand firm – it will change – your new belief will manifest given time and trust.

CHANGING A BELIEF SYSTEM DOESN'T ALWAYS WORK

Nothing happens by chance; The Law of Cause & Effect is an immutable law of the universe. According to the book *The Kybalion*[28]: "The

---

[28] Three Initiates. The Kybalion. A Study of The Hermetic Philosophy Of Ancient Egypt and Greece. Chicago, Ill. The Yogi Publication Society. 1912.

underlying principle of cause and effect has been accepted as correct by all the thinkers of the world worthy of the name. To think otherwise would be to take the phenomena of the universe from the domain of law and order, and to relegate it to the control of the imaginary, something which men have called "chance."

What this really means in our lives is that what we think is what we get. God will not intervene between our thoughts and their effects on our lives. God can only help when we ask for help and are willing to receive the help and recognize it when it arrives. That's why the bible says: *"Ask, and it shall be given to you; seek, and you shall find; knock. And it shall be opened to you."*[29]

What I am writing here is not new. We have read about positive internal self-talk and affirmations for years, from many different sources. But what I have discovered over the years is that no one mentions what I call the "Blips". Blips are, in my opinion, 99.9 per cent of the reason why people give up on trying to change their beliefs and therefore their lives.

> ### *The Law Of Cause And Effect*
> Every cause has its effect; every effect has its cause; everything happens according to law; chance is but a name for law not recognized; there are many planes of causation, but nothing escapes the law. (The sixth hermetic principle from — *The Kybalion – A study of the Hermetic philosophy of Ancient Egypt and Greece by Three Initiates*).

---

[29] Matthew Chapter 7, verse 7. *New American Standard Bible. Reference Edition.* Moody Press. Chicago

WHAT IS A BLIP?

A blip is what the universe throws at you that looks absolutely insurmountable and makes you want to panic. You see it coming and you just throw up your hands and say (to yourself): "All this positive self talk has been a total waste of time, look at what is happening to me, I give up. Life was easier the old way." As a result of this attitude, you go back to being the person you used to be and back to old familiar beliefs and behaviors, because it was easier. You know how to cope and live with the old you. Let's face it – change can be hard.

Why does this happen? I had it explained to me this way when I asked my angel guardians. They said:

"You have spent your whole life building your emotional house a certain way. When you change your belief systems, you have to tear down your old emotional house and build a new house with your new belief system. Sometimes the universe will help you tear down the old house faster by sending in a bulldozer. If you can step aside and let the bulldozer do its job and not stop it, you get to rebuild your new emotional house faster."

Pretty cool I thought. Here's a practical example of what that looks like. My husband and I both had jobs working in the hospital lab industry during the 1980s. During that time period the corporate world, as well as our health care system in Canada, was undergoing a major economic downturn. As a result, a lot of people lost their jobs or were downsized and given new job descriptions. With these new job descriptions came very large cuts in pay and if you refused to take the job, you lost your job to another applicant. It was as simple as that. Everybody had their wages "frozen". By the time we came out of the 1980s we were financially battered and very bruised. We had barely managed to hang onto our house, remortgaging twice just to buy cars so we could keep working. These were years when we didn't know from week to week if we even had a job and it became a joke for us. Every Monday morning we would call each other from work to say, "OK, I am still working, are you?" I remember the day were we were so broke that we couldn't afford to buy the kids ice cream when we went for out for a walk (blip). It was the lowest point in our marriage; we were very unhappy and very stressed out. We prayed that night, "Please help us. Something has got to change."

The following Sunday we decided to go to a different church. We were quite surprised to find that the minister was doing a talk on abundance. She had a lot of very interesting things to say. She talked about negative belief systems and how the universe can only give you what you believe. We went home and took a look at our negative belief systems around money. We discovered the following: my husband, having been raised in a very strict Protestant faith, believed that "you couldn't go to heaven if you were rich" and I discovered that I believed that you "had to be poor to be happy". We were pretty surprised at what our core beliefs were but decided to make a pact to change them to "life is filled with joy, happiness, abundance and prosperity". We knew we had some hard work ahead of us so we promised to help and support each other when the chips were down. And this is what happened to our family over the next six weeks.

We started with our new belief system immediately and within three weeks I was offered a permanent job with a 10 per cent increase in salary (after six years of working three part-time jobs) and my husband got a raise (the first in eight years). We were given a company car so we were able to get rid of our old clunker. Then we had our first blip one week later.

We just happened to come home at the same time one day to find the kids crying and screaming. They were trapped in the basement by boiling water gushing from our water heater. The water heater had literally burst open and hot water was flooding our basement. My husband ran through the water, grabbed the kids and got them out and managed, somehow, to turn off the water supply to the basement. We sat at the bottom of the stairs and looked at all that water; we were devastated.

Now the old us would have said, "See, we are being punished for wanting to get ahead, you are not supposed to want this" but instead we looked at each other and smiled. I said, "Look the universe is washing away our old belief systems." We repeated our new mantra and this is what happened next.

The gas company that sold us the water heater was so shocked at what had happened that not only did they clean up the basement for us but gave us a brand new water heater, free of charge. They had everything professionally cleaned for us and after it dried out there was no damage to the basement whatsoever. The carpets, furniture, and drywall — everything was fine and very clean. No mildew or dampness — anywhere.

Two weeks later we had another blip.

I came home early to find a city inspector in our backyard. He walked up to me and said our chimney was illegal and had to be removed. We had six weeks to remove it or face a $5,000 fine for an illegal fireplace installation. He handed me his card and got into his car and drove off. The whole encounter left me feeling quite shaken and uncertain. We had bought the house with the fireplace and had no idea the previous owners had installed it without a permit. We discovered that it was going to cost $2,000 to have the chimney and fireplace removed and repair the outside wall of our house. We did not have $2,000 but again we just smiled and said, "This is the universe burning away our old belief systems". This is what happened next. My husband found out that even though the fireplace had been purchased and installed by the previous owners, it was still under warranty and we were covered. The company that had installed the chimney came in, made all the necessary repairs, and brought it up to code for a small fee of $500. We could easily afford that because we both had a raise and we had money left over in our savings. The city inspector passed it without incident. We got to keep our fireplace, which we loved and we had money in the bank, which was a first for us.

After these two "blips" life just got easier, more joyful, abundant and happy. We took our first family vacation in years and had a blast. We haven't looked back since and are still amazed at how beautiful life is. We still have the occasional blip around finances but we just smile and know that our new emotional house is built on a firm foundation of belief that life is "filled with joy, happiness, abundance and prosperity".

When you experience a blip it is the universe asking you, "Are you serious?" This is your moment of truth. If you can stand true to your new belief system, then this blip or clearing will get rid of a lot of negative energy in your life very quickly. When you decide to change a belief system remember to stand true to your new mantra.

How To Change A Belief System

I suggest the following procedure to help people rebuild their belief system.

1. Write out the new belief system (mantra) on several small recipe cards.

2. Place the cards around the house where they will be seen all the time. For example: bathroom mirror, dressing mirror, sink, stove, refrigerator, in wallet, on car dash, beside the bed.

3. Every morning the belief system is the first thing you say to yourself and every night the belief system is the last thing you say to yourself. Repeat the mantra every time you look at it. For example: If you are waiting in traffic – say the new mantra to yourself. Repeat the mantra to yourself when you are having any negative thoughts.

4. Keep this up for 40 days. Remember it will take a minimum of 40 days to change a belief system and it can take up to a year for the universe to help you build a new reality around this belief. It is the universe helping you build a new house.

After the 40 days you can choose to deal with another negative belief system that you would like to overcome and select a new mantra or you can continue to use the original one.[30]

Remember, when we change our core negative belief systems we are literally rebuilding our emotional foundation. It takes time to tear down the old emotional house – hence the 40 days – and it takes time to build a new emotional house. But it can sometimes take up to a year for the universe to change what is coming back to you. Remember you have lived your entire life with the old, negative, belief systems and the universe can only give you what you believe. Now you are changing what you believe and the universe has to change what it is sending back to you. This sometimes takes time.

---

[30] Hay, Louise. "I Can Do It. How To Use Affirmations To Change Your Life." California. Hay House Inc. 2004.

CHARLENE
OVERCOMING PANIC ATTACKS USING ENERGY WORK

Are we being of service to teenagers when we try to medicate them with antidepressants? Here is a story of one young woman who overcame panic attacks that immobilized her to the point where she stopped attending school.

In the spring of 2003 Charlene began to suffer panic attacks. She began to notice increased periods of anxiousness and shortly thereafter began to suffer periods of unconsciousness and fainting. The fainting spells could occur at any time, under any circumstances, but they were primarily occurring while she was in school. Over time the fainting began to occur in social situations and eventually resulted in her fainting at home when she was resting or walking around the house. Charlene's mother said that her overall wellness seemed to be a factor as they noticed she would faint more when she had a cold or the flu.

Her doctor examined Charlene and numerous blood tests were done. All results were normal. Her doctor, being very thorough also ordered an ECG, EKG, heart monitoring, CAT scan and a MRI. Again all tests gave normal results. Charlene was beginning to have increased periods of fatigue and feelings of listlessness. She was already under the care of a chiropractor and he had not found anything out of the ordinary that would explain her periods of anxiety or fainting spells.

Charlene was referred to a therapist and by the time that I met her, she had been in talk therapy for over a year. There was no noticeable improvement, her feelings of anxiety were becoming more pronounced and it was decided by her heath care team that a period of rest from school for a semester would be in order.

Charlene came to the Paradigm Centre in the winter of 2006. She was 17 years old and had been off school since the previous June. She presented as a quiet, well-behaved young lady. She was well groomed but walked with her head down and her voice low and soft. She was anxious and wouldn't make eye contact. She said that her therapist and her physician had referred her. She told me that they were thinking of putting her on anti-depressants and that she might have to go into the Homewood to work with her anxiety. (The Homewood Health Centre specializes in treatment programs for people with mental illness.) She didn't want to do that. She was afraid, she said and didn't want to take drugs. She wanted to know if I could help her. I said we would see; I couldn't make her any promises because energy work depended on her willingness to heal. I also explained to her that with energy work I could only walk beside her on her path. Energy work doesn't do anything the mind can't handle or the body will not accept. I explained to her that it would take some time, but how much time would depend on her, where she was willing to go and how she handled the work and how often she did the sessions.

In the initial appointment we reviewed her current family history. Charlene explained to me that she began to have panic attacks when she was 15. She found Grade 9 to be a difficult transition and only had one best friend in high school at the time. She had loved grade school and felt that the first six years of school were some of the best years of her life. When she moved to middle school she found it hard because the teachers there weren't very nice to the students and "treated us all very poorly", she said.

Charlene said her childhood was normal and she was very happy. She was really close to her mom, brother and dad. She said that she loved camping and playing cards with her dad, her brother could be a pest sometimes but they got along well most of the time and that her mom was her best friend. When she was little she had lots of imaginary friends, was good at keeping herself occupied, played well with others and had lots of friends at school.

When I examined Charlene's aura you could immediately tell she was an Indigo[31]. Indigo children are highly intuitive, sensitive, extremely creative and can be very independent. Indigo children have a tendency to view the world with a different pair of eyes. They see the world in all its many forms. They need to experience the world in a creative, tactile way, which means that they learn by experience, touch and sound. They can read people very quickly but are easily confused when they begin to understand that the world does not treat them with the same respect and understanding. This often leads them into thinking negative things like: "something wrong with me", "I am weird", "nobody understands me". As a result they often suffer from anxiety, panic attacks and will withdraw into the safety of their home life or friends, or unfortunately, if the first two options are not available to them, they develop addictions in order to self medicate or tune out.

I asked Charlene if she knew what an "Indigo" was. She told me she had heard of them and always wondered if she were one of them. When I

---

[31] Indigo Children have a natural ability to sense, feel, or know another person's feelings. Because they are so sensitive to their environments they often react to other people's emotions but don't understand how to distinguish between their feelings and the other persons. They are often labeled ADD, ADHD, or suffering from Anxiety or depression.

explained to her how they see and experience the world, she got tears in her eyes and said, "Yes, that is what I feel." At this point Charlene took a deep breath and began to relax physically. Her energy field opened up and I was more easily able to "see" what we were dealing with in her situation.

After Charlene lay down on the table we began energy work. First I ran my hands over her energy field to feel the flow. We gently worked with the body's innate wisdom to uncover and remove blockages to her emotional and physical fields primarily in the chakra of self-esteem or third chakra.[32]

When we were finished I explained to Charlene that she might feel really tired or really jazzed. If she was tired she needed to rest. She was not to kid herself about the level of fatigue and she may feel like a bus had hit her. She may be weepy or sad. She was just to rest, let herself cry, or if she felt moody to write or draw out her feelings. She needed to drink a lot of water and be careful driving, as she may feel lightheaded for a day or two. I told her that the clearing would subside within 24 – 48 hours. I also explained this to her mother so that she would receive additional support if this did happen.

Two weeks later Charlene reported that she felt really good for a week but then the past week had been all downhill. She said her anxiety had increased and she felt depressed.

I told her that this type of reaction was quite normal and was an indication that the body was accepting the changes and beginning to heal and release. She said she "knew that" and was quite comfortable

---

[32] Chakra is Sanskrit for "wheel" and signifies one of seven basic energy centres in the body. Each of these centres correlates to major nerve ganglia branching forth from the spinal column and is related to physical and emotional components.

with the process. In this session the body identified blockages in her hormones and reproductive organs.

At her third session, one week later Charlene reported that she "felt really good". I noted that when she arrived for this session her head was up, her eyes were brighter, and she was making eye contact with me when she spoke. With the body's wisdom and permission we worked on feelings related to "always feels like a 5th wheel" and fears of "never fitting in". Her body was dehydrated so we worked with balancing out body hydration and we discussed the importance of drinking lots of pure water.

I did not see Charlene again for five weeks due to holidays. When she arrived for her session she said that she had returned to school. She told me that she "was apprehensive" but was "doing OK". In this session we continued to work on emotional blockages related to her intuitive feelings around "don't want to offend my parents", "fear of expression", "who am I", "don't know who I am", "confused about life" "something wrong with me", "I am different". We spent a lot of time talking about free will and the free will of others. We talked about different coping strategies on how to deal with her intuitive feelings and how it applied to her everyday life. We also discussed what to do with those feelings.

Children who are highly intuitive are naturally energetically empathic so it is very easy for them to pick up on other people's feelings and fears. If they don't understand how to distinguish between what they are feeling and what the other person is feeling, they begin to think it all belongs to them. They start to have what they commonly refer to as "crazy thoughts" and "can't understand where these thoughts come from". They interpret this as "their problem" and "there is something wrong with me" and "no one will understand and think I am crazy". But once you teach an Indigo or intuitive child how to separate their feelings from other people's feelings, they calm down dramatically and begin to understand what to do about them. They learn how to be conscious of their own feelings and recognize that they have choices about how they respond to the world around them.

At the eighth week of sessions Charlene said things were going well. She certainly gave every appearance of looking like it was. When she arrived she looked like a different person; I almost didn't recognize her. She walked in confident, head up, sharply dressed, her hair was nicely done, her voice clear and articulate with direct eye contact. She looked quite stunning. We worked at clearing emotions from her mother's past. These were subconscious emotional layers that Charlene carried in support of her mother and was totally unaware of their existence.

This again often happens with Indigo/intuitive children. If they feel another person's pain, they will often pick it up and carry it in their own field out of love and devotion for another. This weighs them down because they don't know what to do with it and leads to confusion because they can't understand why the other person doesn't suddenly get better. As a result of this energetic exchange they begin to feel "useless" or ask, "Who am I?" or say, "I don't know who I am". This begins another cycle of anxiety, depression or panic because they don't know what to do next.

We discussed the importance of loving another enough to let them learn how to "walk" with their own emotions. I explained to her that her mother trusted her enough to learn how to walk when she was born, so she should learn to "trust" her mother enough to figure out how to handle her own emotional issues. This means energetically, allowing her mother to feel her own issues and if Charlene was concerned for her, then to practice the art of "sending love". We also discussed some energetic emotional guidelines that I had developed over the years as a result of working with highly intuitive people.

They are:
1.   Just because you know, doesn't mean you do.
2.   Wait to be asked.
3.   Do only what is asked.
4.   If you are not asked and you are concerned, just love them with your heart.
5.   If you feel another person's emotions enter into your field, you have the right to choose to let that emotion go.

At Charlene's ninth session she reported that things were going well at school. She said she was still having problems with fainting spells so we asked for and received permission to work with the physical body. We worked with balancing out the body's ability to deal with sugar. I asked her to follow a sugar free (and no artificial sweeteners) guideline for two weeks. I have also found over the course of working with intuitive children or Indigos that they are very sensitive to sugars, artificial sweeteners, wheat, and additives. If they can be encouraged to follow a natural, wheat free diet and drink water and natural fruit juices it is much easier for them to cope physically and emotionally.

As we balanced out the physical body we talked about coping mechanisms for Indigos. Indigos easily connect to fear, especially when projected by others. As a result of their ability to connect energetically to other people's emotions they begin to fear that they created the fear in the first place or are at least responsible for fear. This will again cause them to withdraw and become overwhelmed with emotional responsibility. Parents unfortunately magnify these feelings when, in their efforts to protect their children, they tell them all the things they can't do, or shouldn't do but fail to explain what they can do or how to handle a situation if it should arise.

We talked about understanding how the world does not need to be a scary place and how to use your intuitive abilities as a coping mechanism. We worked through some practical applications of different social scenarios and I showed her different ways to use her intuitive abilities as well as the "energetic emotional guidelines" to think her way through a problem.

When you show Indigos how to use their intuition instead of being afraid of it, they quickly see that they have options and choices. They begin to naturally choose very practical solutions and then don't find the outside world so overwhelming. They learn that what they are feeling is valid. What they are feeling is true for them. They learn how to separate their feelings from another person's feelings and yet still retain their enormous capacity for love and empathy for themselves and others without being overwhelmed and fearful.

It is important to remember that Indigos experience the world around them in a tactile way. Once they are taught how to use their intuitive gifts in relation to how they feel, they very quickly learn how to "feel" their way through any type of problem. They learn how to think on their feet. When this happens they relax and demonstrate how highly motivated, intelligent, loving, and empathic they truly are.

Charlene knew that she didn't need to take drugs to solve her panic attacks and anxiety. Thankfully, her parents, doctor and therapist supported an alternative management method, namely energy work. In this case, therapy included: clearing chakra energy blockages; helping her understand her own thoughts and feelings; clarifying her emotional responsibilities as well as enhancing her diet.

Charlene returned to school after being off for six months. At the time of publication Charlene had finished high school and was preparing for University. She demonstrated a sense of confidence, power and joy as she prepared to tackle her future.

The Art of Sending Love

Thoughts and feelings create vibration. The Art of Sending Love teaches you how to use the truth of that statement to help another person. It is a simple technique of thinking about the person you are concerned about and then saying to them silently, in your mind as you think of them, "I love you." We know for a fact that this technique works by testing the size of a person's energy field before and after they have been sent thoughts of love. To test the truth of this use dowsing rods. Have a friend stand at one end of the room. Take your dowsing rods and measure the size of their field. Remeasure the person's field while the person is thinking angry thoughts. Now repeat the test while the person is thinking loving thoughts. Look at the difference in size of their measurements. Have the person go back to thinking an angry thought and you think of them and then say: "I love you." Remeasure the field. I think you will be most surprised at the result.

For an explanation of dowsing rods see the Glossary.

HOW DID ENERGY WORK HELP CHARLENE?

Charlene suffered from panic attacks, anxiety and fainting in spite of the fact that all of her tests were normal. She tried talk therapy, chiropractic and traditional medicine and finally came to energy medicine as a last resort.

Energy work helped Charlene to identify that she was an intuitive, who sensed and felt the world around her. Charlene, during her sessions, became aware of the periods of transition in her life that had impacted her emotionally. She learned different coping strategies that allowed her to deal with her intuitive feelings and gave her the ability to apply them to her everyday life. As a result Charlene was able to make the emotional transition of loving and accepting herself. Charlene overcame her panic attacks and anxiety and her fainting spells disappeared.

Rae
Strengthening Emotional Boundaries

Rae is a homemaker who has a good life. She has been happily married for over 40 years and has always loved being at home with her children. She gets a lot of joy out of her grandchildren and frequent visits with family and friends. Rae grew up on a farm during WWII with her mom and grandparents while her father was away at war.

She loved the farm and felt the first five years of her life were magical. When her father returned from the war life got sad. Her father and grandfather didn't see eye to eye and a short time later the young family moved away to the city to start a new life. She missed her grandfather because she always felt like he was her real dad. When her father returned from the war, "He was a wreck. He was really emotional and had bad nerves," Rae said. He never sought any professional help because in those days "you just didn't do that." Life wasn't easy and the family was always short of money.

Rae married young and had her children quickly. Life was good but she developed heart problems early and had been on some form of blood pressure medication for most of her adult life. When Rae first came to the practice she was suffering from sleep apnea, high blood pressure, hemorrhoids and was overweight. She was hoping she could get help with her weight and maybe start to sleep better because she didn't like the breathing machine, that much.

When I first looked at her aura there was a large fear cord with her father. It was settled primarily over her heart and lungs. We removed that. After we were done, the body asked for and received balancing to her overall energy field, which we call "*Laterality*". The body then asked for additional balancing on her heart, lungs and overall circulation system.

When Rae returned to the office a few weeks later she told me that for the first time in her life her hemorrhoids were all gone. She was thrilled. She also found that she felt calmer and that the energy work was helping her. She asked if we could work on some emotional issues that had been a problem regarding her son and his partner. We did fear cord removals with both of them. The body then requested more physical work and we did a balancing with her body on how it metabolized sugar, protein, and water and then we balanced the thyroid. I told her that as a result of the sugar balance she needed to eliminate all sugar from her diet for two weeks. I explained that she could have all the fruit, vegetables and meat that she wanted but no sugars or artificial sugars. She needed to drink a lot of water as well.

When she returned a month later she said that the month had been a challenge because of the sugar balancing. But what surprised her was how quickly her blood pressure had come down. Rae said her doctor was thrilled and had recommended she reduce her blood pressure meds. She wanted to know if we could work with her body around blood pressure and help her get it back to normal. We asked for and received permission from the body to work on blood pressure. The body surprised me when it asked her what she wanted her blood pressure to be. I had never heard of this. When I relayed that piece to Rae, she didn't hesitate for a minute, she just said, "Oh good, I would love to have it around 118/80." Body agreed.

Body then went into diastolic pressure first. Here we found an emotional block that formed around the age of 18. Rae told me that when she was 18 she didn't see eye to eye with her father and he was always hard on her. She never felt like he was really her father, because her grandfather had been "her dad" for the first five years of her life. Her dad was "always worried about what other people thought." After we cleared this block from the emotional level of her field we uncovered another fear cord. This one was from her grandmother that developed as a result of her constant worry about her son overseas, at war.

A month later when Rae returned, she said that the last month was a "weepy" time for her. She had been thinking a lot about her life at age 18 and remembered how it was such a sad time for her. Rae also said that currently there were some problems between her husband and his friend. Her husband's friend had married a friend of hers and they had recently split up. "They were some of our closest friends and the divorce has been really hard on me," she said. I asked her why? She said: "I feel responsible for their marriage, if I had never introduced them, then this would never had happened. It is all my fault. My husband and I are the ones everyone comes to and then we get dumped on for helping."

After some further discussion I asked her if she felt she was ready to work on "taking responsibility for other people's emotional responses." Now normally when body wisdom makes an emotional statement like this, this is where we work, in the emotional field. We would look for causes of the belief, when it originated and then work at clearing a core belief. But the body went into the physical instead and asked to have the liver, kidneys and lungs balanced. As always, following body wisdom, despite what we felt emotionally to be the right thing to do, we did as asked. When the body was done balancing, her field oozed and cleared layer upon layer of worry.

Rae came in for a second session an hour later. (This is not uncommon as clients travel great distances and will do up to four appointments in a day.) At this session the body went back to "worry" and we uncovered a belief that "I have done something wrong," and "What would the neighbours think?" These two statements originated at age six. Rae remembered being in school and always "trying to be a good girl".

At her next session an hour later, the body went into the lungs and here we uncovered more childhood beliefs and fears around "no one wants me" and "I have to be perfect." Her aura released mucoid strands of resentment and worry off her abdomen and lungs.

Over the next few months we continued to work with her body requests for balancing with lungs, circulation and kidneys. During this time period Rae began to uncover belief systems on her own and would come into the sessions with statements she wanted to work with. She couldn't get over how much calmer she felt. She still needed the meds for blood pressure and was still on the breathing machine to sleep at night but she felt better about her life over all and was quite intrigued how all of her belief systems seemed to be working together. Rae was on a roll and ready to tackle more.

When Rae returned a few months later she said she had been for a stress test. She said that it had come up in our last session together and that I had recommended that she see her doctor and have one done. I had no memory of that but I always trust what the angels guide clients to do. She was glad she had gone because she had been feeling a lot of pressure in her chest and was getting tingling in her arms and right leg. The doctor said that her stress test had some abnormal results and that if she had any more symptoms she was to get to the hospital immediately. "Well, that really got me worked up," Rae said. "I just sat there and stewed about that all day and all night. The next morning I felt awful and told my husband you better take me to the hospital, something doesn't feel right." Rae was admitted immediately and for the next two days the hospital ran tests. All the tests came back normal and the doctor said to her, "You just keep everything inside" and felt that she was suffering from anxiety. Rae said that really woke her up.

She really wanted to work on what she kept holding inside. Over the course of her next sessions, the body kept returning over and over again to age six. Rae said it was one of the most difficult times in her life. She had spent her whole life on the farm with adults and animals. Then one day she finds herself standing in a schoolyard filled with children she never knew existed. Up to this point in her life she had always been told she needed "to be a good girl." She knew what that meant at home but at school, what did that mean?

At the next session the body took us into her parasympathic system and found the whole story at age six. The body's wisdom showed us how at age six she was expected to be a good girl and "do as you are told" but no one was telling her how to behave at school. This revealed her belief that "no one loves me and no one ever tells me what to do" and "that it is not alright to do as you want".

When these statements were repeated back to her, her field opened up a short movie.[33]

I saw a little girl sitting at the table learning how to make pies with her mother and grandmother. I saw the Grandmother turning to her and saying, "You have to be a good girl at school; you have to do as you are told". She looked confused and you could feel her thinking about what that meant. The movie stopped.

Rae said yes she remembers being in the kitchen with her mom and Grandmother and how they would teach her how to make pies. Her Grandmother was very strict and was always telling her and her mom what they could and could not do. Rae said by the time she got to school she was afraid to do anything.

At this point another movie opened up:

I saw a little girl in a schoolyard. She is shy and standing to the side of the school, there is dirt and grass under her feet. She watches the other kids running around laughing and playing. No one comes and talks to her. The movie closed.

Rae said she often spent recess standing by the wall and watching the other kids play. She was afraid to play with the other kids because she didn't want to ruin her clothes. There wasn't a lot of money and you had to make do with what you had, she said. At this point the psyche of the body's wisdom at age five said, "Never ask, never told."

---

[33] See Glossary

Rae said this was so true for her. She was never allowed to ask questions, but she didn't trust herself to know the answers herself. Everyone around became the outside authority. Because she was raised to be a good little girl and do as she was told, she often found herself in situations doing what she was told even though it felt wrong and made her unhappy.

"Now that you remember what it was like for you as a child, what if some of the people closest to you are going through the same feelings and emotions? Now that you know how you felt, what if you took that information and used it? You could start to understand how they would react to something and then ask yourself: "What would I have liked to know if this happened to me? Could that bring about a change for you?

As a result of this, Rae began to trust her inner feelings and developed confidence in expressing them. She was able to take her natural ability to empathize and see situations from the other person's point of view and stopped taking responsibility for the way they acted. This helped her to feel more comfortable socially, she became more relaxed emotionally with her family and her blood pressure started to come down. Her physician is currently in the process of reducing her blood pressure medication.

How Did Energy Work Help Rae?

Rae was a homemaker who loved her life but years of struggling with high blood pressure, sleep apnea, hemorrhoids and her weight left her feeling desperate. She decided to give energy medicine a try.

Energy work helped Rae to identify and remove several major fear cords that created energetic interference in her heart chakra. Her diet was adjusted and sugars reduced. This allowed her body to heal from hemorrhoids and her blood pressure started to come down but it did not completely resolve the problem.

Further energy work on the emotional levels clearly showed Rae how her need to be "a good girl" had led her to believe that she was "responsible for other people's emotional well being". Once she was consciously aware of how her beliefs were affecting her emotional health she was able to make the necessary changes to her belief systems and adjust how she reacted to other people's emotional well-being.

Rae's blood pressure continues to improve but does increase when she is emotionally upset. She is now aware of how to handle the emotional component and is working with her doctor to reduce her blood pressure medication.

PETER
OVERCOMING OBSESSIVE COMPULSIVE DISORDER

Peter is a 55-year-old male and father of four. He presented with obsessive-compulsive disorder, sleep apnea, irregular heartbeat and lipomas[34] He had tried numerous therapies over the years and had little success. His obsessive behaviour was beginning to affect his job and he was concerned that it was preventing him from advancement within the company. Peter had seen how successful energy work had been with his children and their allergies and was very motivated to see how energy work could be of assistance to his compulsive behaviour.

Peter and I have never met. He receives all of his energetic treatments by distance work as he lives elsewhere in North America. We only worked together for about three months.

In this particular session when he arrived energetically, the body requested that we focus on the lipomas, which cover his body. Although the intent in his sessions is to deal with obsessive compulsive disorder I have learned that the body will sometimes take you to an area that at first seems totally out of the realm of what is needed. But if you trust its voice you often uncover a core issue that is acting as a block to the healing requested by the client. When I acknowledged body's request to focus on the lipoma, I heard my guide, the Archangel Michael say:

"Blocks to self- love."

---

[34] Lipomas are benign tumours composed of fatty tissue.

When I told Peter this he paused and felt that it was not an issue. I said, "Let's see where it takes us." At this point the body's energy field shifted so that I was focusing on his jaw. I was taken into the jawbone and then into his immune system. When I arrived inside the immune system at the point of the energetic obstruction the following information was given to me by the body and I heard the statement: *Self hate – past life.*

At this point, the body started up a *movie*. The movie showed me a past lifetime of his where he is a priest. *The priest is lying in a bed and his surroundings are simple and very drab. He is cold, weary and it feels as though little is being done to attend to his needs. It becomes obvious to me that he is in his last few hours of life and has been left to die in peace. As he lay there his thoughts are being relayed to me. He is looking over his life and realizing how he had lived a life of quiet desperation. He felt like his life was a failure; his reasons for entering the priesthood were selfish and self-serving. He had spent his life hiding behind the walls of the monastery and behind God. He felt that his life would have been more complete if he had entered into the world, married and had children.*

At this point the movie stopped and I was returned to the area of energetic block inside his immune system. I was not asked to release the blockage at this point, only to acknowledge its presence. I honoured and related the movie as seen, uncensored to him. After this information was relayed to Peter, the body shifted my focus into his heart chakra and here the body showed me another energetic blockage that stated the belief system *no right to exist.*

I was told that this belief system was also a result of this past life experience. Peter became very choked up at this point. He said that he often felt that he didn't like himself very much and he wondered what was the point of his existence. He never understood where these random feelings came from. With his acknowledgement of these feelings, the heart chakra opened and I was given permission by the body to release that blockage using a combination of Therapeutic Touch™ and chakra balancing. As the blockage lifted I heard the Archangel Michael say the following and I relayed this to Peter:

"Belief that he has to be significant and save the world. He is angry that what he does is not important enough (self judgement) and therefore he drives himself and others forward in order to attain his need for importance."

Then Archangel Michael instructed me to relay to Peter:

"Look at the importance of loving kindness to others and to himself and understand that this is all God expects of him is love. Love of himself and loving others. Peter, when you can turn to the person beside you and love him in non-judgement - you have attained perfection."

At this point I could sense the blockage fully lift and clear, and as it drained the heart chakra balanced and opened. The body then indicated to me it was full energetically and requested that the session be closed.

A short time later I received this email from Peter:

As always, I appreciate your treatments and the information you pass on to me. I believe what is surfacing is right on target. I am not sure if you have had the opportunity to read the Power of Intention by Dr. Wayne W. Dyer. I was reading Dr. Dyer's book and on page 44 two topics appeared: "Kindness toward Oneself" and "Kindness toward Others" just after receiving your treatment and report. His book is reinforcing the message from Michael the Archangel. In addition, I have modified recommended affirmations to personalize them and saying them has also been beneficial. I am confident that the treatments are working.

A short time later Peter emailed to say that his lipomas were decreasing and that his obsessive-compulsive behaviour was becoming more manageable. He had recently been promoted and he was finally able to move his family back to their home state, much to everyone's delight. When he was ready to continue, he would contact me to do further healing.

How Did Energy Work Help Peter?

Peter had an obsessive-compulsive disorder that interfered with his career. He also had lipomas and sleep apnea. He had tried everything in an effort to overcome his disorder and heal his lipomas, which were spreading.

Through the process of energy work his body revealed a past life belief that affected his heart chakra and manifested physically through his lymphatic system to create lipomas. When the past life beliefs of "self-hate" and "no right to exist" were brought forward into his consciousness, he knew that these feelings had been playing out his entire life. He just never understood where they came from.

Peter chose to work with these belief systems and change them. He learned how to love himself and appreciate who he was and what he had to offer. He began to understand and live the truth that his existence was important. Within six months his obsessive-compulsive disorder became more manageable and his lipomas decreased. As a result of these changes in his attitude toward himself, Peter was more productive at work and received a promotion.

KEVIN
CANCER OF THE BRAINSTEM

When Kevin was first brought to my office he was five years old and had been given six months to live. When he came to see me he was unable to walk or speak; he was pale, thin and unable to sit by himself. His parents brought him to me for comfort measures and had no expectations for recovery or a cure. Kevin had been through a lot in his short life and had suffered a great deal.

His parents explained to me that Kevin had been diagnosed with a brain tumour (medulloblastoma) earlier that year. He underwent surgery to remove 98 per cent of the tumour. He then underwent six weeks of radiation therapy followed by a chemotherapy program, which was halted after six weeks because they found new tumour growth further down the brain stem. The doctors had told them that there was a new tumour and that there was nothing more they could do for him. They recommended a course of treatment that could possibly prolong his life but the prognosis was poor – Kevin had about six months left to live.

At this point the parents decided to halt all invasive therapies and to continue only with non-invasive holistic therapies to make his life as comfortable and painless as possible. The family had just returned from a final trip to Germany – a gift from the "Make-A-Wish Foundation.®"[35] Kevin had ongoing issues with vomiting, lack of balance and hearing loss

---

[35] Make-A-Wish® Foundation Canada is part of the largest not-for-profit wish granting organization in the world, serving 30 countries with international affiliates on five continents. Since inception in 1980, Make-A-Wish® has helped make over 200,000 wishes come true for children around the world.

due to the surgeries and medical therapies. His condition was being monitored monthly at a prominent children's hospital in Canada.

As Kevin's parents told his history, I felt as though time had stopped in the room. I was stunned – I had never worked with a child who was dying. I was afraid that this situation was way beyond my capability to be of good service. I immediately consulted with my angel guides and asked, "Who should I refer them to?"

Archangel Michael said,

"They have been referred to you for a reason."

I responded, "But I don't have the experience or the expertise to help them."

"Why do you think they have been sent to you? Because you can help.

You are not alone.

We are here to help you with this most precious child.

Be still and know God."

This gave me the courage and confidence to continue with the session. I explained to Kevin's parents that I could only walk beside their son on his healing journey and that there couldn't be any guarantees. The parents were aware of this and felt that if anything could be done to ease their child's suffering then it was worth it. I remember being struck by their calm demeanor, their patience with Kevin and with me. And I realized that they were at peace with whatever needed to happen. They were here as advocates for their son and they were going to do whatever that child needed at whatever cost, because they loved him and they were willing to honour his journey wherever it needed to go.

I suggested a schedule of treatments and we decided to do them mostly by distance work as Kevin needed to be carried everywhere and because his family had to travel a long way to my office.

At every session I would connect to Kevin's brain stem, locate the tumour and work energetically in that area. After that I would go to the body as a whole and balance whatever was requested to help it with the overall healing. We continued this course of work twice a week over the next four months.

During this time Kevin's parents also worked with a local doctor of traditional Tibetan medicine and incorporated custom designed nutritional supplements created by the Canadian Cancer Research Group and a nutritional supplement available commercially call IP-6. They also adhered to a strict diet that was sugar free that included organic foods and juicing.

At each session I would see Kevin's body and view it at an energetic level; I would focus in on his tumour. As a medical intuitive and HET, I am able to visualize the body at the cellular level and see what's going on and find out what needs to be done. I continued to work with the tumour to dissolve it and helped the body to eliminate it.[36]

---

[36] For more information on this form of energy work: *Adam. DreamHealer: A True Story of Miracle Healing*. Penguin Group (Canada), a division of Pearson Canada Inc. 2006.

The tumour appeared as a creamy white mass running down his brainstem and behind his left ear. It was soft to the touch, thick and had the consistency of fatty tissue. The body was oblivious to its presence and this really surprised me. It was like a parasite that had attached itself to the brainstem and the body was compensating and working around it instead of trying to fight the tumour.

I also noticed that the tumour had an off-key hum to it. In my experience when I work with the body I sometimes perceive organs energetically in an auditory fashion such as humming. I know an organ is out of balance when the hum is off-key. I've also discovered that when an organ goes off-key, the body will initiate an immune response to correct the problem. (For example if there is an infection in the lungs it will create a different tone in that organ and this helps the body to initiate an immune response to fight the infection.) But in this case it wasn't happening. This was unusual.

The body seemed to be seeing the tumour as if it was a normal organ. And even though the tumour had an out of sync hum to it the body was not initiating an immune response (trying to fight the tumour). I was uncertain what to do with this information at this point so I continued to focus in on the physical aspects of dissolving the tumour energetically.

Over the course of the next four months the tumour began to shrink in size and became more opaque. At one point I thought it was completely gone but was hesitant to say anything to Kevin's parents because I didn't want to create false hope. In my training as a healer we go into every session with a blank slate with no expectations. This way we are open to what the body is trying to say. We don't interfere with outcome or project our ego issues onto the body. When I went in and couldn't find the tumour, my first reaction as a healer was that I had somehow wanted so badly for this child to get well, that I had projected these results. I felt it safer to wait for medical confirmation that the tumour was gone.

During the four months of energy work, his parents reported that Kevin was demonstrating dramatic and incremental improvements. He started to gain weight, was beginning to walk again, and was vocalizing more. On occasion, Kevin and his parents would come into the Paradigm Centre for his sessions. One day I was overjoyed to see that Kevin was climbing the stairs to the treatment room with little assistance. Shortly afterwards I received a call from his parents asking if they could have my permission to release my name to Kevin's oncologist at the hospital. Kevin's father explained to me that when they took Kevin into the hospital for his monthly testing the oncologist had to review all the tests twice because they couldn't find any trace of the tumour. He knew that they had done everything medically possible and the tumour had started to grow back. Now the tests were showing it was gone and they had no explanation for it. The doctor was amazed and wanted to know what the parents had been up to with Kevin. The parents said they would tell the doctor but only after they had received permission from the healing team, who had been working with Kevin.[37]

Kevin, by this time was also beginning to display rapid improvement to his balance and hearing. By the summer of the next year he was walking on his own with little help and his hearing was almost 100 per cent. His

---

[37] Although I gave permission to do so, to this day I have never been contacted by the hospital or the oncologist to see if this treatment could be of assistance to other children.

response time to events was improving and he continued to gain weight and was growing again.

As we continued with his course of treatments his eyesight continued to be a concern as he had little control over eye movement, making reading difficult. Kevin's parents decided to bring him into the office for this session.

After he was comfortable on the table, I asked for and received permission from his body to work on his eyesight. Using the Medical Intuition Body Scanning technique[38], I entered through the iris of the eyes and traveled back into the primary optic nerve centre. Standing behind the optic nerves I was able to observe that the electrical pulse to the right eye was out of sync with the left. The eyes were unable to move in concert with each other, making focusing difficult and erratic. After continued observation of how the electrical impulses were moving through the optic nerve I was able to isolate which electrical bundle was damaged. Moving into the bundle, I observed how the neurons looked tangled, burned and were soft to the touch. I compared these neurons to other neurons in the optic nerve that were healthy and could see how and why they were unable to communicate with each other.

I moved into one of the neurons and asked body if a correction was done here could the body translate the correction along to the other neurons. After receiving permission, and using energy work techniques, the neuron was repaired. I waited as the correction was translated outwards and when I received confirmation from the body I placed my energetic hands on the back of each eye and moved them to see if they would move in concert with each other.

---

[38] Medical Intuition: Lori Wilson's Total Body Intuition ™ Technique

At this point Kevin threw up his hands and held them in the same position as I was holding my hands inside his head energetically and began to move them in concert with me. He yelled out, "Whee!" We all laughed. Once I was sure that the correction was complete I withdrew my energetic hands from behind his eyes, Kevin dropped his arms to his sides as I withdrew. Within two weeks both eyes were beginning to show dramatic improvement with hand to eye coordination moving along nicely. Kevin's parents were overjoyed that he was beginning to read again and could return to school.

Five years later I was honoured to be contacted by Kevin's family. They asked if they could come for a visit and interview me for a book they were writing about Kevin's experiences. I laughed and said it would be wonderful to see them again and I was just in the process that week of drafting an email to them asking if I could interview them for my book. The Lord works in mysterious ways.

It was a joy to see Kevin again. He had grown to be quite big and was managing well on his own. His reaction times were still slow and walking was still a little awkward but his overall demeanor was of health and vitality. I was glad for this rare opportunity to see him post treatment and find out how he was.

After five years of being cancer free I asked his parents how Kevin was doing. His father responded that in general he was doing well. His energy level was better, his speech was coming through more fluently, his eyes were fine, he was walking better and they were seeing improvements every few months. His mom often noticed that before he improved there was a plateau and some regression – either emotional or physical. I have found that this is a common occurrence in how energy work progresses.

His father went on to say that Kevin was never going to be at the same level academically and socially as other kids his age but was very physically active. He had been doing martial arts for a couple of years and was doing very well. Although he loved school, Kevin often felt isolated and lonely and this continues to be part of his ongoing journey.

I asked his parents about Kevin's memory. His father said it was generally very good but when he was tired his memory would start to fade as would his physical body. He explained that the oncologist told them that when Kevin had the surgery they had cut through the cerebellum and they are only now starting to realize that the cerebellum has a lot to do with unconscious processes. So things that you and I do automatically – like riding a bike – we don't have to think about, but when Kevin does these things it requires a lot more energy because a lot more of his vitality has to go into focusing on them.

I asked his parents if Kevin was still being monitored by the hospital. They told me that because he was over the five-year mark, he was now in a long-term care program with a team that included monitoring by oncology, neurology and psychology. They continued to do tests and in the spring of 2007 Kevin had had an MRI and everything was fine.

His father said: "If you were to ask the oncologists they would say he is doing well. And that is what they are saying – unexpectedly well."

I asked Kevin's parents why they decided to turn to energy work. Energy work is very new in terms of people's beliefs and understanding of healing. It's a whole new paradigm that people are still trying to figure out. Here's what Kevin's father said:

> "We had talked about this and I don't think we were expecting too much. We had been told the worst – we were told that our son was going to die! And I remember that I was crying and grieving for days. I had never been to an energy healer before and I thought let's see what this is. There was this overall feeling of openness and lack of anxiety but it was also very emotional because I think it was about accepting death. And I think that we were both emotionally and spiritually mature enough to look at those issues. But I was willing to accept the fact that our son might die. And once you do that, you know there is that old Native American saying, 'It is a good day to die'. You just learn to face that and it becomes a part of your life – and it takes courage. And I think that both of us found courage. So there were spiritual forces that we were able to access and were guiding us at that point. I do believe that."

And this is often the case in my practice. This is a classic example of a family that took advantage of everything that traditional medicine had to offer and ran out of options. But somehow they knew that there was something more that could be done. Turning to Tibetan medicine when Kevin was a baby and had an untreatable cough for six months was one of their first steps to having proof that complementary health care can work. It is like prayer. You are never really sure if it will work but you try it and are thrilled when it does.

It is interesting to note here that Kevin always looked forward to his sessions at the office. His parents said that he enjoyed being on the table and the "do dabs" (filters) that I used. He found the work to be "a little adventure." This is the beauty of working with children – they have no preconceptions and are happy to go along and see what happens.

Kevin's father made a very important statement about the role of parents in healing a sick child: "I think that as parents you have to advocate for your child. In terms of the healing process we went through with Kevin, he saw that we were doing all of these various things, and he realized that we were on his side. And we were showing him that he was worth the effort and that gave him the confidence that he needed to get through this," he said.

Because this family was so new to the concept of using energy work, I asked Kevin's parents when they started to notice a change. Was it after the first session? Was it after a couple of months?

They both said that after each session they would notice that Kevin would be more balanced, a little clearer in his energy in terms of what he was doing and how he was functioning. Overall they found the sessions produced results that were fairly noticeable, yet the improvements were subtle.

Because they were working with several different forms of complementary health care, they said that Kevin was on a massive healing trajectory and that made it hard to discern which treatment created which result.

As a healer I run across this conundrum all the time; trying numerous types of healing modalities at once but not being sure if any one modality in particular, was the one to heal the problem. This is because people are used to a patriarchal[39] medical model where you do one thing or take one pill to solve the problem. When you pursue complementary health care you are entering what I call a matriarchal[40] healing model. This means that you may need to do several healing modalities together, in order to produce the change. In the end it does not matter what you did or in what order, what matters is that you are getting better. This matriarchal medical model is much more intuitive. Not all illnesses are physical and nor are they all emotional. There can be an interaction between the physical, emotional and spiritual aspects. All aspects need to be addressed in order to assist in healing.

Kevin's father recounted a story about Buddha that I love: "When you see a guy lying in the street bleeding to death you don't run and get a medical text book. You want to deal with the problem and help him heal – not figure out intelligently what caused it."

How Did Energy Work Help Kevin?

Kevin was diagnosed with a brain tumour and sent home to die after surgery, radiation and chemotherapy failed to stop its growth. His parents brought Kevin to my practice for comfort and had no expectations for a cure.

Energy work, in combination with Tibetan medicine, nutritional supplements specifically designed for Kevin, along with a natural organic, sugar free diet helped Kevin to recover from inoperable cancer.

---

[39] See Glossary
[40] See Glossary

Kevin and his parents loved their son and realized that they had to become advocates for him. With courage and faith in their son's will to live, they reached out and expanded beyond the normal medical paradigm and achieved what many believed to be impossible – a miracle. They helped their son to heal from cancer.

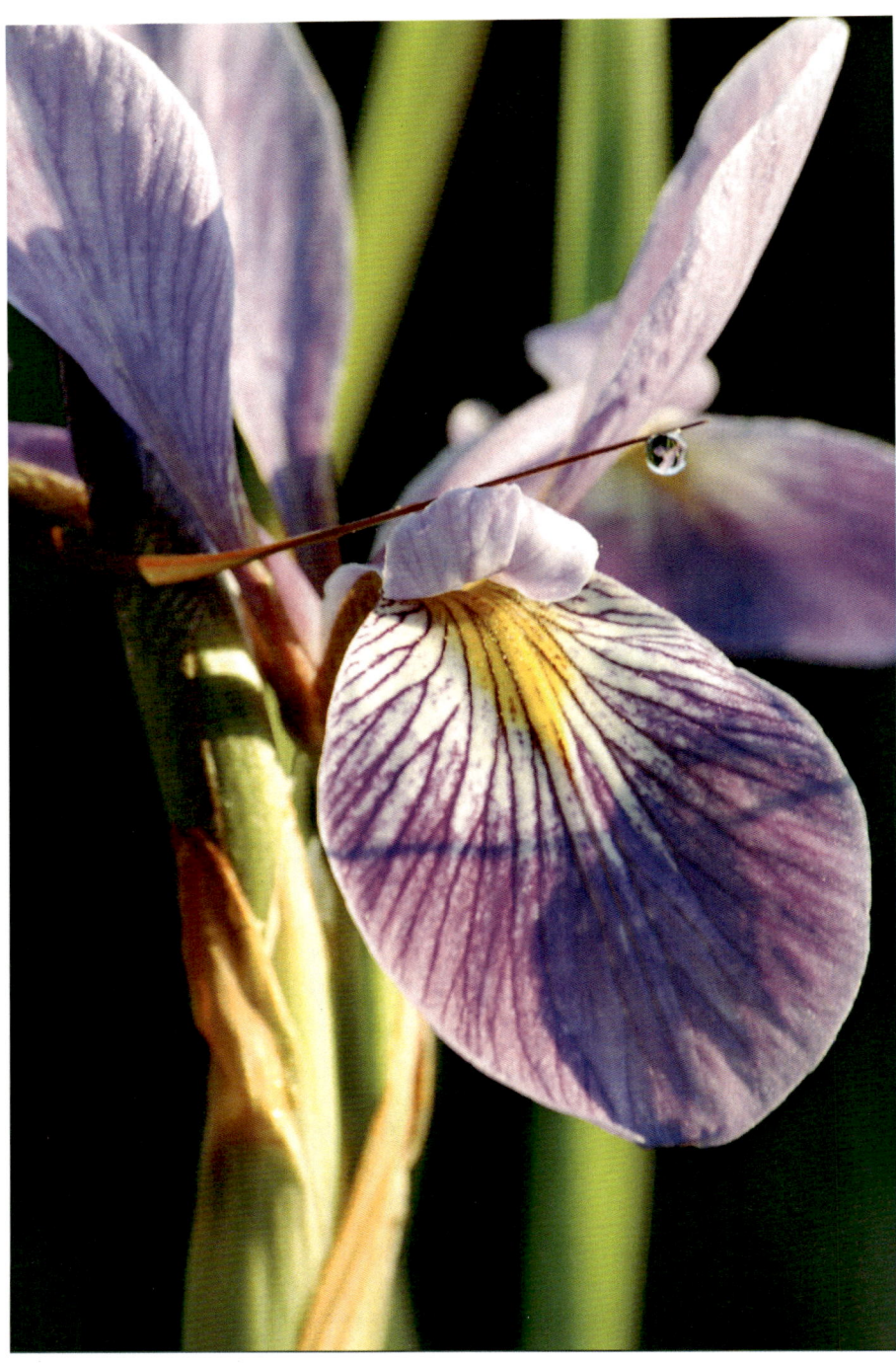

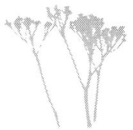

GUIDELINES FOR WORKING WITH A HOLISTIC ENERGY THERAPIST

You have decided to work with a Holistic Energy Therapist (HET) and do energy work to help resolve your current health issues. What should you expect and how do you take care of yourself during and after a session?

First of all, remember that you have gone down into the valley of un-wellness which means that you are suffering symptoms of one kind or another. These symptoms can represent energetic blocks in the energy body or aura. These energetic blocks can be on a physical, emotional, mental or spiritual level. When you undergo sessions of energy work, your body will be moving through these levels to release energetic blocks.

What does this mean? It means that there might be a reoccurrence of symptoms but the symptoms will never be as bad as they were when they first started to appear. Eventually you will back out of your original symptoms and return to health which is not a linear process. Clients may experience this as one step forward and two steps backward and often feel frustrated. At this point some clients stop their sessions because of their confusion about the process. Energy medicine practitioners call this process of moving through symptoms a healing cycle with valleys, peaks and plateaus.

VALLEYS, PEAKS AND PLATEAUS

When clients experience a healing cycle with valleys, peaks and plateaus they become increasing aware of their symptoms and begin releasing their energetic blockages. This is a process that isn't always comfortable or easy.

The valleys are a part of this healing cycle. In the valleys symptoms can resurface, appear to be worse, or just show up again after being gone for several years.

The peaks are an absence or reduction of symptoms.

Plateaus are new levels of health, wellness or feeling better overall. Plateaus can last an hour to weeks, months or years.

In essence I explain energy work to all my clients this way. Energy work can be subtle or dramatic. Your body has gone down into the valley of un-wellness and energy work will be bringing you up out of that valley. This means that there may be a reoccurrence of symptoms. The symptoms will never be as bad as they were when they first started to occur but they will be there. How your body responds to the release of these systems can be subtle or dramatic. You may feel tingling, coolness, heat or trembling or the sensations may be more dramatic and you will feel the need to cry, moan, or feel angry. In some extreme instances clients need to scream. I explain to clients that how the body "chooses" to work through the original symptoms may not be logical because the body will not do anything that the mind cannot accept or the body cannot handle. In other words, the body wants to heal, it does not want to feel pain. It will do whatever it has to do to go back to the place of peace and harmony but it will do it in a way that is safe for it because the body does not want to re-traumatize itself. Whatever the body is feeling we need to allow that feeling to express itself.

- This means that if you feel the need to cry – you cry.
- If you feel the need to sleep – you sleep.
- If you feel the need to pace – you pace.
- If you are feeling angry – feel angry.
- If you need to be alone – be alone.

Find a safe way to feel and allow the body the experience so that you can understand what the body is trying to tell you.

IF YOU FEEL THE NEED TO CRY

If you feel the need to cry and want to cry but are worried about how people will respond, cry in private. My personal favourite is having a long hot bath, a cup of tea and a big fluffy towel to sob into. If by chance my children heard me and got worried I would just tell them, "It is OK, mom is just having a good cry." This helped my kids feel safe, and taught them it was OK to feel sad sometimes. My husband liked it because I wasn't trying to take my sadness out on him or, trying to make him responsible for how I was feeling.

If you are a man and don't cry, that is OK too. Go for a long drive. Take a walk. Go fishing. My husband travels a lot and personally likes the freedom of being left alone in a hotel room to do his personal processing. I like that because then I don't get all worked up and start thinking it's my fault and he is unhappy about our relationship.

If You Need To Sleep

Go to bed. The body does a lot of deep healing in the sleep state. Worried about dinner? Order in. Tell the kids you need to sleep. Take a nap in the middle of the day. Go to bed early. Sleep in. Take a day off and sleep all day. We have all heard the statement, "Things will look better in the morning." They usually do and things will get better.

If You Need To Pace

Pacing can be a great way to work out what is really bugging you. If you find that there was a statement that came up in your energy work session and it is really bothering you might want to try this. Keep repeating the statement to yourself over and over again. What are you feeling? What do you think about? What memories are coming up?

A few years ago I received a call from my sister. We were just having the usual sisterly chat when she made a casual statement about a family party that I hadn't been told about. I went absolutely ballistic. Thankfully I felt it coming and didn't say anything to my sister (because this wasn't about her) and made some plausible excuse and got off the phone – pronto. I put down the phone and realized I had a really rich opportunity to figure out why I was reacting so badly to that statement. I wrote down exactly what she said. This is called a "trigger" in energy work. I then started to pace back and forward repeating the trigger statement over and over again. And I just let myself be livid. I cried, I stomped and I just kept walking back and forth, repeating the statement over and over. When my husband asked me what I was up to I just said, "I've got some healing work to do here, I will be fine." He said, "OK" and left me alone.

(It is important to be left alone here and not start making this all about everything else.)

After about 10 minutes I remembered something that had happened when I was 16. It was a memory of not being included in a family gathering. I got angry all over again. I continued pacing repeating that story at age 16 over and over again. About 15 minutes later I remembered being five years old. When I was five, my sister and I had the same best friend. My sister got invited to her birthday party and I did not. I was suddenly five years old again and I remembered how angry and deeply hurt I was. I let myself cry and cry. Afterwards I felt a whole lot better and learned something new about my feelings and myself around my family. I always felt excluded but realized that I had excluded myself because of a belief that I took on at age five. I changed that belief.

IF YOU FEEL ANGRY

Find safe ways to be angry. Yelling at the telemarketer, the kids, your spouse or the dog, does not solve the problem. You are feeling angry and you need to find out what causes that anger in you. The only way that will happen is if you let yourself feel the anger, talk to your anger and let your anger show you what is making you fearful. Anger is just an expression of fear in its extreme form. The sooner you let yourself see what you are afraid of, the sooner you will have a grip on your anger.

Safe ways to deal with anger can be: taking long walks, journaling (I like to use a red pen and scribble a lot), pacing out the anger incident, hitting a pillow, pulling weeds, raking the leaves, working out or cleaning.

IF YOU NEED TO BE ALONE

Find a room, a corner. Be alone with yourself. If you are worried about how your family will respond, tell them you need some alone time. I call it the "I love you but..." response. I love you but I just need to be left alone for a little while. So long as the people around you don't feel like they are the problem, they will be quite happy to let you do your thing.

When I began my training as a healer I was still working my corporate job. It was a difficult transition because I was working in a physical world but developing my spiritual faculties. I found that the only way I could cope and keep my sanity moving between these two extreme worlds was to have lots of alone time. We had a small bedroom in our home that wasn't being used regularly so I took it over. I painted it and put a bed in there and a small bookcase. I moved all my spiritual books in there. Every morning I would get up a little early and go to "my room" and meditate. When I got home from the office, I would make dinner, clear up, make sure the homework was OK and then go into "my room". I would read, listen to music, journal, cry, stare at the ceiling or just let myself feel. I told my family what I was up to (I call this *processing*) and when I shut that door, no one bothered me. In my home a closed door means privacy and we all respect that.

Let's now apply these principles to someone who is having problems with joint stiffness. Aaron is a middle-aged computer tech who woke up one morning to discover that his left thumb was swollen. He thought it was probably because they had been moving a rather large piece of equipment the day before at the office and thought nothing of it. Over the next five years the stiffness came and went. He always put it down to moving something or lifting something. As this progressed he started to notice that he felt stiff in the mornings when he woke up. Again he put it down to physical activity. Maybe he was working out too much and needed to ease up a little. He used lighter weights, shortened his work out times, and varied his workouts. The stiffness continued to progress. One morning he couldn't get out of bed he hurt so badly. He saw the doctor who started him on meds for stiffness and told him he was getting older and that he was probably starting to develop arthritis.

Aaron started to think that he had arthritis and took the meds. After time the meds didn't work and he needed a stronger prescription. After a short period of time they didn't work either. He started to take supplements that helped arthritis. It worked for a while and then all his symptoms came back with a vengeance. He was perplexed and frustrated. At the urging of a friend he started to see me for energy work. He didn't understand it but felt he was desperate and had nothing to lose. (A common response, skepticism and disbelief.)

As we started energy work he noticed that there was instant relief from his symptoms of stiffness and joint pain but what surprised him as we worked through his sessions, was that he started to have problems with acid reflux. He said that he used to have that problem when he was in college, years ago but it eventually went away after taking antacids for a few years. He thought it was because he was under a lot of stress at school. When he graduated, the problem went away, confirming his belief that the acid reflux was stress related. We continued with the energy work and he took the occasional antacid between sessions but after a few more sessions the acid reflux went away. This is great, he thought. (Now he was a believer, energy work is helping).

One morning he woke up and couldn't move. He thought he'd had a relapse, and was afraid that the energy work was making his symptoms worse. (Very common situation, people start to believe that energy work harms, not heals and will often discontinue their work with an energy worker here.)

He came in and talked to me about it. I explained to him again that as he heals there will be a reoccurrence of earlier symptoms. I asked him if the overall body stiffness was as bad as it was the first time it happened. He said no, it wasn't but it reminded him of how bad it had been and he was afraid of it coming back. This is quite normal I told him and after the session he felt a whole lot better but he told me he could tell he was feeling really, really angry. I asked him if he knew what he felt angry about and he said he wasn't sure and wanted to think about it. "That is totally OK," I said. Aaron didn't come back for a couple of weeks. When he did come back he told me that he had taken a long drive and just let himself feel the anger. He was surprised at what came up. He said that he found he kept saying to himself "nothing ever goes right" over and over again. And it made him so angry. He remembered a lot of different things in his life that fit that belief and had spent the last several weeks thinking about it but he felt he was missing something. (Now he was understanding how to use energy work for himself and let the process of feeling his emotions show him what to do.)

I had him focus on the statement "nothing ever goes right" and then let the body show me where it was sitting in his body. The large intestine meridian came up. When I tapped into the flow of the large intestine meridian I could hear crying and feel abdominal pain. I saw the image of a small baby and a mother pacing back and forth. I could hear the child crying. I could hear the mother saying, "Nothing ever goes right." I asked Aaron if he knew if he had colic as a baby. He said he didn't know but he remembered his mom telling him that he could never sleep at night and that she would give him an aspirin when he went to bed and then he would sleep. I asked him about this belief "nothing ever goes right" and if that made sense to him. He said, "You know it does. My parents were new immigrants and they had a really tough time when they moved here. They were always saying that to each other."

At his next session Aaron told me he had a chance to talk to his mom about his childhood and she told him that he did have colic as a baby but they didn't know that at the time. They couldn't speak English, none of the other kids had that problem and his mom was afraid she was doing something wrong with him and "nothing was going right". Times were hard for the family when they first immigrated to Canada and everything frightened them. This made sense to Aaron and coincided with how he felt about things as a child when he was growing up.

When Aaron returned for his next session he told me, "You know since we started working on this memory my bowels have been acting up again."

I asked, "Again?"

"Yeah, I always had diarrhea when I was a kid. I had totally forgotten about that."

Again we have a reoccurrence of an old symptom. This symptom was originally a problem in childhood, long forgotten because the body couldn't get his attention, so it found another way. It had moved to acid reflux in college.

We worked with diarrhea in the bowels and the body moved our attention up into the small intestine. I asked him if he had ever been tested for food allergies. He told me he had not. I suggested he get tested.

When we got the test results back Aaron found out he was lactose intolerant. He never knew he was allergic to dairy. I find that babies suffering from colic are having an allergic reaction. Mothers are often told that their baby is allergic to their breast milk but in reality both mother and child are having an allergic reaction to the same thing – in this case dairy. Aaron made the necessary dietary changes and within three months his muscle and joint stiffness was gone, his thumb got sore every once in a while but he told me, "I know that when it hurts, I have cheated and had some dairy. As soon as I stop eating dairy, my thumb is fine again."

After all the work Aaron had done with energy work, this is a synopsis of what the underlying problem for him was. As a baby Aaron had colic. Because his mother was under so much stress after moving to Canada she couldn't breast feed him like she had with all her other children. He was put on cow's milk. Because his parents "felt nothing goes right" he probably "drank in" this belief every time he was fed.

When you look at Aaron's developmental timeline, this is what is revealed. As a baby, Aaron suffered from colic, as a child he developed diarrhea, as a young adult, acid reflux and as an adult, muscle stiffness. As Aaron got older the muscle stiffness developed into joint pain. As he healed, he started to back out of the original symptoms. In energy work we call this a *"healing cycle"* or *"going down into the valley of un-wellness"*. For Aaron his healing cycle manifested as a temporary increase in joint pain that moved into muscle stiffness, which cleared into acid reflux, which moved back into diarrhea, which lead to the discovery that he had a dairy intolerance. When he eliminated milk products from his diet his physical symptoms cleared. Each healing cycle lasted from one hour to three days. After the cycle was over, his symptoms would settle down to something he could tolerate. We call this a *plateau*.

He continued to take care of himself in the plateau. He let himself feel the emotions, dealt with the discomfort by taking his medication as prescribed and the supplements he had chosen. This eventually led to him coming off medication and taking the occasional aspirin to deal with the discomfort. Aaron's healing took approximately one year to overcome his symptoms while undergoing energy work two to three times a month depending on his symptoms, how he felt and what his schedule would permit.

This is a practical example of the secret to energy work; walking through the process and learning how to take care of yourself.

As I stated earlier in the book, we forget the body is a living, breathing organism. It feels. It feels through sensations. These sensations can be pleasure or pain. These sensations will "trigger" emotional responses in the mind. The body can only talk to you in symptoms or feelings. If you don't listen to it, eventually it will find another way. It will keep looking for another way to get your attention until you have a crisis.

In his book, *A New Earth: Awakening Your Life's Purpose,* Eckhart Tolle talks about the pain body and states:

"Any negative emotion that is not fully faced and seen for what it is in the moment it arises does not completely dissolve. It leaves behind a remnant of pain."[41]

Energy work goes into those symptoms or "pain body" and helps you to find out what exactly the body is trying to tell you. It is as simple as that.

Energy workers or HETs act as interpreters for the body. We read body language and then help you understand what to do about it.

In the example with Aaron, we see a classic case of a child who has a physical problem that became attached to this parents' emotional distress of "nothing ever goes right" (developed a pain body). When he was able to remember and understand that belief system, he was able to move back to the original cause (being lactose intolerant) and he healed from his physical symptoms (released from the pain body). At an emotional level, it put his life back into context and he is currently in the process of re-working his belief systems.

Whether you do *the work*[42] or not is up to you. A holistic energy therapist can't make you heal. That would interfere with your free will — something even God won't do. But a holistic energy therapist can walk beside you, as an interpreter and help you to read the signs, remove the blocks, free the energy and thus give the body the freedom to heal.

The rest is up to you.

---

[41] Tolle, E. (2005). *A New Earth. Awakening to Your Life's Purpose.* United States: Penguin Group.
[42] Energy work, body work or releasing blocked energy

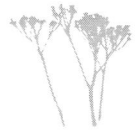

UNDERSTANDING A HEALING SESSION

The principle of energy work is to help you to heal physically or emotionally by clearing blocks from your energy field or aura by using different *modalities*[43] or techniques.

You should expect to be processing for 24-48 hours after a session. This means that you need to take care of yourself by resting, attending to your emotional needs and drinking plenty of water.

Some of the terms that you may hear in a session are *tracking* and *scanning*.

TRACKING

In energy medicine when we do tracking, we are in fact following an energetic string that can go back in time to determine when the blockage first occurred or solidified into conscious belief. For example, during an energetic scan of the body, the body can reveal a blockage in a chakra. When contact is made with the blockage in the chakra the body can make a statement that demonstrates a belief such as "lost myself". When I encounter these statements I will ask the body wisdom, "Is there an age of attachment?" If body says, "Yes" I will ask, "What age?" Body will then state an age or I will muscle test what age it occurred. When I muscle test for what age it occurred I start with:

---

conception, in-utero, birth, age one to five etc. until the correct age is located. When the correct age is located I will ask the client: "Do you remember any incidents at age X where you began to believe 'lost myself?'". The client will think and often go to the correct memory at roughly the correct age. I then have the client stay focused on the memory and then have body wisdom show what needs to be cleared in the energy field as a result of this memory. Often it is an organ or organ system that is holding the blockage. When this blockage is cleared, the client releases the memory.

Scanning

Scanning refers to the holistic energy therapist taking her hands and running them over the energy field. The hands are held about one to two inches off the body and then using a sweeping motion, the hands are swept down over the body and limbs. This technique, similar in style to Therapeutic Touch™, also finds irregularities (called blockages) in the energy field. Blockages will indicate an area that the body is trying to bring to attention. A HET will pause and sit with the blockage. I call this listening energetically to feel what the body is trying to relay in relation to the presence of the blockage.

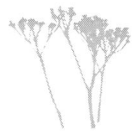

TRAINING

If you are considering training in the healing arts, I would like to take this opportunity to dispel any myth that I suddenly woke up one morning and "knew" how to do healing work and opened a practice. Some are born with this gift. I was not.

I was gifted with being more open to my intuition than most because my parents were both psychic. They recognized my intuition and taught me to be comfortable with it and not to be ashamed. This made my eventual training extremely easy.

When I finally acknowledged my intuition it was the result of two young men who "saw" what I could do and then encouraged me to get the right training. Both of these lovely young men, continue to this day to be my mentors and teachers. They are Russ Mater, Craniosacral therapist and Larry Steel, B.O.S.™ Practitioner at the Steel Health Centre. Larry introduced me to a young woman who is a pioneer in helping others to develop their intuitive abilities and to channel and use the tool of Medical Intuition with integrity and ethics: she too continues to be one of my advisors; her name is Lori Wilson[44]. She has founded Inner Access 101™, an Education and Resource Network which offers specialized training in Channelling, Regression, Medical Intuition and Business Intuition. All of these colleagues are superb leaders in their fields.

---

[44] www.inneraccess101.com

There can be a difference between a holistic energy therapist, healer, energy medicine practitioner and someone who does laying on of hands. Each title depends on their training, certifications, background and beliefs. I am a holistic energy therapist who practices energy medicine. It is what I choose to call myself based on the numerous modalities that I have trained in.

My training is never done; I continue to learn every day. I am instructed by my angel guides but I have also taken extensive training with the following teachers and modalities. I invite you to visit their websites and learn more about energy medicine and what it has to offer.

Biocomputer Operating System™ (B.O.S.)   www.steelhealthcentre.com

Total Body Modification™ (TBM)   www.tbmseminars.com

Medical Intuition: Lori Wilson's™
Total Body Intuition™   www.inneraccess101.com

Intuition & Channelling Higher Wisdom™   www.inneraccess101.com

Age & Past Life Regression   www.inneraccess101.com

Angel Therapy Practitioner® (ATP)®   www.angeltherapy.com®

Craniosacral Therapy   www.russmater.tripod.com

Therapeutic Touch™   www.therapeutictouchontario.org

If, after reading this book, you have made the decision to pursue a career in the healing arts I encourage you to consult and research any or all of these modalities. You may also be interested in my next book which will review the basics of an energy medicine practice. This is information that I believe healers should know and understand in order to run and manage their own successful practices and to be of ethical and integral service to their communities.

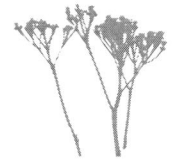

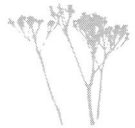

ACKNOWLEDGEMENTS

This book is the result of urging from my guides, the Archangels Michael and Gabriel. The book was proposed in a meditation when I first opened my practice ten years ago. My angels suggested that I write about what was happening during a healing session. They explained to me that the public could use some guidance about energy medicine and what happens in an energy healing session.

Over the years, I would often hear them comment during a session, "This is for the book." I shared this with a colleague one day, and I openly pondered if I really had the ability to write the book and if it would ever really be published. My colleague just said, "The book will write itself." She was right, it has.

When you decide to leave a successful career to follow your dream, it helps to have someone in your life who isn't afraid to let you try it out. As a result, my practice and this book would not have happened without the love, courage and constant support of my husband, Bert. When I told him I was quitting my corporate job to open a private practice, he just looked at me very calmly and said, "OK, but promise me this, if you haven't got any clients in three months, will you go out and find a real job?" Five years later we danced through the lobby of a century-old home we bought because the practice had grown too large to remain in my home.

When I first started my training as a healer my kids were surprised, but they thought it was pretty cool. To obtain my certification I had to learn and practice the healing modalities. Willing participants were needed and my daughter quickly recruited her many friends. Each night I would come home from my day job to find my daughter's friends sitting in the family room waiting to be "worked over" as they called it. They would all hang out and watch movies while I meticulously worked through all the techniques I was learning. They were great and I learned a lot. I give my heartfelt thanks to my daughter Jessica and her cornucopia of dear friends.

My son was the most laid back of everyone and said little in the beginning of my training but if he wasn't feeling well, he was always the first in line to get balanced. I have many fond memories of all six feet of his lumbering frame standing over me while I lay in bed in the early morning saying, "Mom, I need a balance." Adam, you never hesitated in believing in me. Thank you.

When my training was completed additional volunteers were needed in order to complete my certifications. Twenty brave souls volunteered and gave willingly of their time. They were patient and had the courage to go into their healing with full trust, when I was still training. It was a rich time of discovery and to each and every one of you, my deepest gratitude.

As my practice grew I needed help booking appointments, answering the phone and looking after clients when their sessions were over. To my assistants over the years, Andrea Munk, Kristen Mandzuik, Melissa Koschmider and Shelly Mast, thank you. Getting the book done in its finally stages, would not had been possible without the coordinating talents of my current assistants, Ellen Taylor and Amanda Griffin.

For over five years my personal assistant Isabella D'Alessandro provided me with invaluable support, not only managing the office, but also my life, always with gracefulness and love. Thank you for taking such good care of me and my clients.

Three years ago I met a young mom, Susan Bushell. Little did I know at the time what an impact she would have on my practice. She asked me if I would train her. I had never even considered training anyone. I was not sure I was ready to take on a student but she had it all worked out and showed me how I could teach her. The Angels just smiled broadly. That was the beginning of my mentoring and training of Apprentices. My students and I thank you for opening the doors of knowledge.

My healing abilities would never have been awakened if it had not been for my teachers and mentors. To Russ Mater, Larry Steel, Lori Wilson, Andrea Matheson, Sandi Loytomaki, thank you for helping me see my innate abilities and hone them with integrity, efficiency and due diligence.

This book and the work would not be possible without my clients who allowed me the honour of being of service. I continue to walk into the treatment room daily and be in awe of your courage to find your own truth and it is an honour to be of service on your inner journey.

The Paradigm Centre for Wellness, the centre where I work and has been my dream, would not have not been possible without the patience and hard work of two very gifted business advisors, James Nagy and Karie Huisman. Thank you for helping to make this dream a reality.

To my dear friends, Christine Johannink, Susan Bushell, Patty Oser, Sharon Hall, Judi Bechard and Pat White, for their love, warmth, laughter and always being there with just the right words of support, the perfect book or the presence to just have a night out and go to a movie when things got crazy: I am grateful for your help in remembering that we intuitives are perfectly normal, every day people, who happen to have a different view of life.

The creative aspects of this book are the result of the artistic talents of Dr. Bruce Walton, a dear friend and mentor. Bruce took me under his wing and has been a valued advisor. His calm and patient perspective, as well as his uncanny ability to look at the other side of things has been invaluable. I am honoured to include his amazing photography. It is the perfect complement to the message of the book.

This book would not be possible were it not for the editing gifts of J. Kundan Abelsohn. Her ability to guide this book to its completion has been enhanced by her intuitive abilities and understanding of the healing arts, being a talented clinical aromatherapist herself. She has been a gift to me from my angels.

My work is a tribute to my guides, the Archangels Michael, Gabriel, Raphael and Ariel, our Lord Jesus, and Mother Mary. I am deeply grateful for their daily presence, guidance and teachings. They teach me every day. It is my honour to be in their presence and a student of their teachings.

Namaste,

June 2009

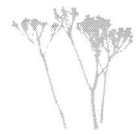

GLOSSARY

Affirmations Statements of belief. For more information read: *You Can Heal Your Life* by Louise Hay. (See references)

Allopathic The system of medical practice which treats disease by the use of remedies which produce effects different from those produced by the disease under treatment. MDs practice allopathic medicine. Also called conventional medicine.

Astral Body Also referred to as the Astral plane, it is a bridge between the spiritual and physical bodies.

Aura An electromagnetic field around all living things. Human beings have the most complex energy field and it is comprised of four major layers: physical, emotional, mental and spiritual. These four levels are also referred to as "subtle bodies". It is perceived as a light or luminous body that moves around the physical body.

Balance Another term for a healing session.

Biocomputer Operating System™ (B.O.S.)	B.O.S. or Biocomputer Operating System is an innovative energy harmonizing technique that taps into the body's inborn potential to heal itself. For more information: www.steelhealthcentre.com
Brain Gym®	Brain Gym® is an effective training program that helps to overcome learning challenges by using 26 specific repetitive movements, which help to create new pathways in the brain. For more information: www.braingym.org
Celiac Disease (CD)	"Celiac disease is a medical condition in which the absorptive surface of the small intestine is damaged by a substance called gluten.

This results in an inability of the body to absorb nutrients — proteins, fats, carbohydrates, vitamins and minerals — that are necessary for good health.

Although statistics are not readily available, it is estimated that one in 133 persons in Canada are affected by celiac disease.

A wide range of symptoms may be present. Symptoms may appear together or singularly in children or adults. In general, the symptoms |

of untreated celiac disease indicate the presence of malabsorption due to the damaged small intestine."

Official definition of celiac disease from the Canadian Celiac Association.
For more information: : www.celiac.ca

Chakra
Chakras are Sanskrit for a wheel and signify one of seven basic energy centres in the body. Each of these centres correlates to major nerve ganglia branching forth from the spinal column and is related to physical and emotional components.

Chakra Balance
Technique to balance the chakra system or individual chakra.

Christ Light
Also called universal healing light, spirit light, God light, Divine love, healing light etc. In healing work there is a rule that when something is removed energetically from the body's energy field, you cannot leave a vacuum. This vacuum is always filled with divine healing light and speeds up body healing. Healers are trained specifically to do this is in a grounded, heart centered and loving way to assist with the body's healing.

Crown Chakra   See Seventh chakra

Distance Work   Distance work is the ability to work with a person's energy without being physically present with that person. Distance work is done over the phone at a pre-arranged time or it can be done at any scheduled time and results called or emailed to the recipient. Healers "dial-in" to the person's energy field and then work with their energy. It is similar to listening to the radio and tuning into a particular station. Distance work can only be done with the client's verbal or written permission.

Dowsing   Dowsing is the art of finding hidden things such as water or magnetic fields. Usually, this is accomplished with the aid of a dowsing stick, rods or a pendulum. Dowsing is an ancient practice whose origins are thought to date back at least 8,000 years.

Dowsing Rods   Dowsing rods can be made of wood, copper, brass or even coat hangers.

Ego Body   The ego body is created in our consciousness during infancy and is based on our sensory experience of our bodies. It forms the belief that we are distinct from other objects. Energy work helps bring to conscious awareness that the ego-body boundary is only a mental construct.

Emotional Body

Holds our emotions and feelings

Emotional Freedom Technique™

EFT™ is an emotional version of acupuncture that stimulates certain meridian points by tapping with your fingertips. For more information go to: www.emofree.com

Energy Medicine Practitioner

Also called a healer or energy worker. They practice the healing arts and act as interpreters for the body's innate wisdom.

Energy Therapy

A form of healing art that acts as interpreter for the body's innate wisdom. Can be practiced by energy workers, energy medicine practitioners and healers.

Energy therapies can be identified as energy modalities.

Energy Work

Energy work releases blocked energy in an auric field. If left unchecked, it can eventually manifest in physical, emotional or spiritual symptoms.

Energy Worker

Also called a healer or energy medicine practitioner.

They practice the healing arts and act as interpreters for the body's innate wisdom.

Etheric Body

Holds the energetic template or blueprint for the physical body.

Fear Cords

Energetic representations of fear. They appear as cords coming out of the body. They can vary in texture, colour, size, depth, thickness and emotional nature. Most often found between parents and their children. Usually produced by the client or accepted from another with whom they have a strong emotional connection. Fear cords are very easy to remove either by the client themselves or with assistance from a healer.

Fear Snakes

A deeply rooted fear that energetically appears in a tubular or string like shape. This form of energy has often been carried since childhood, or has been carried on the soul path as the result of a past life trauma.

Fifth Chakra

Also called the throat chakra. It is situated over the throat area and represents how we communicate with the world.

First Chakra

Also called the root chakra. Lies at the base of the tailbone and represents how we stand in the world.

Fourth Chakra

Also called the heart chakra. It is located in the heart area. It represents how we love.

Gas Distribution Visualization (GDV)

Stimulated electro-photonic glow around human fingertips that contains very accurate information about the state of the person's health. For more information go to: www.kirlianreasearch.com

God Source

For the purposes of this book I refer to God but readers can substitute spirit, the divine, source, universal consciousness or any other word that describes a higher power. I have a tendency to refer to God in the male gender even though I experience God as being "The All" – both male and female.

Healer

Also called an energy worker or energy medicine practitioner. They practice the healing arts and act as interpreters for the body's innate wisdom. Healers are intuitives who can see, sense, feel or hear energy fields or auras around all living things. A healer is a student of this energy and learns what the different patterns, colours and shifts mean. Healers learn how to clear stagnant or blocked energy in an aura by training in numerous modalities or remembering an innate knowledge. They just know how to heal without understanding the "why" or "what" of it and just follow their instincts or intuition.

Healing Journey

Journey of awareness and experience that helps a person who is unwell find their path to wellness.

Healing Miracle

When the client and the body recall what created the block in the first place and release it. Symptoms abate and there is peace and harmony, emotionally, physically and spiritually.

Healing Team

Any practitioners, traditional or complementary that you choose to work with. Also a term used if there are more than two healers working with a client at the same time.

Healing Wheel

Looks like a wagon wheel. The hub in the middle represents the individual. Each spoke of the wheel represents a healing practitioner (alternative or traditional). Each spoke added to the wheel gives it additional strength and provides momentum. The client decides what is to be included inside the wheel and how the wheel will move forward.

Heart Chakra

See Fourth chakra

HET	See Holistic Energy Therapist
Holistic Energy Therapist (HET)	Holistic Energy Therapists or HETs are intuitive healers and energy workers who practice energy medicine. They have been trained in numerous modalities. They are often trained as medical intuitives.
Indigo Children	Indigo Children have a natural ability to sense, feel, or know another person's feelings. Because they are so sensitive to their environments they often react to other people's emotions but don't understand how to distinguish between their feelings and the other persons. They are often labeled ADD, ADHD, or suffering from anxiety or depression. To learn more read: *The Care and Feeding of the Indigo Child* by Doreen Virtue. (See references)
Intuition	The Canadian Oxford dictionary describes intuition as: the power of understanding situations or people's feeling immediately, without the need for conscious reasoning or study.
Intuitive	The Canadian Oxford dictionary describes intuitive as: characterized by or possessing intuition.

Kirlian Photography   Is a photographic recording of the faint corona discharge induced by the application of a high voltage but low current electrical field to an object which is in direct contact with a photographic material. http://encyclopedia.jrank.org/articles.

Laterality   A term used by B.O.S. practitioners to describe a particular balancing technique. This technique was developed by Dr. Harvey Steel and Larry Steel. It balances right brain with left brain and improves memory, speech, concentration, and balance.

Mantras   A word, statement, or sound repeated for meditation or to change an old belief system.

Matriarchal Healing Model   Looking at the body as a whole, at all levels, energetically. (Author's definition)

Medical Intuition   This is a tool of supplementary insight. It traces the nature and roots of conditions that have manifested themselves in physical discomfort and disease within a client's energy field. For more information on Medical Intuition: www.inneraccess101.com

Medical Intuitive   They use their intuitive abilities as a tool of supplementary insight and trace the nature and roots of conditions that have manifested themselves in physical discomfort and disease within a client's energy field.

Mental Body

Processes and holds our ideas, thoughts, and beliefs about who we are in the world.

Modalities

Term used by healers to describe what they have been trained and certified in.
Examples of modalities are:

- Therapeutic Touch™
- Reiki™
- Biocomputer Operating System™ (B.O.S.)
- Total Body Modification™ (TBM)
- Body Talk™
- Acupuncture
- Chakra balancing
- Chinese medicine
- Emotional Freedom Technique™ (EFT)™
- Homeopathy
- Herbology
- Polarity Therapy™
- Bowen Technique™
- Craniosacral therapy
- Clinical Aromatherapy
- Healing Touch™
- Naturopathic medicine

For a more complete list refer to: *The Subtle Body. An Encyclopedia of Your Energetic Anatomy* by Cyndi Dales (see references)

Movies

In energy work we find that the body will "play" what we call "movies." They are short, visual and "seen" through the third eye. They can be symbolic of what the body is trying to say or they can be an actual replay of a memory. Movies are relayed to the client by the HET and the client determines whether the story feels right or true for them.

Muscle Testing

Is a form of biofeedback that tests the muscular strength of a client. Muscular weakness indicates that an imbalance and muscular strength indicates balance.

Muscle testing also responds to simple yes/no questions. It is also referred to as Kinesiology.

New Paradigm or New Healing Paradigm

Energy medicine, working in conjunction with allopathic medicine. (Author's definition)

Past Life

A life lived prior to your current lifetime. Based on the belief in reincarnation.

Patriarchal Healing Model

Symptom based healing model. Looking at and treating for symptoms. (Author's definition)

Physical Body   The physical body that we see, feel, touch and experience. The physical body also holds seven primary chakras, twenty-two secondary chakras and about thirty-three thousand tertiary chakras.

Processing   Honouring what you and your body needs after a energy session or balance. Sleeping, crying, feeling sad, angry, or read, listen to music, journal, stare at the ceiling or just letting yourself feel.

Psychic   The Canadian Oxford dictionary describes psychic as: "a person considered to have occult powers, such as telepathy, clairvoyance inexplicable by natural laws." Psychics predict the future (Intuitives do not predict the future.)

Quantum Physics   Quantum physics is the study of the behavior of and at the molecular, atomic, nuclear, and even smaller microscopic levels. It has been determined that quantum particles do not follow the same laws as larger molecules.

Root Chakra   See First Chakra

Second Chakra   Also called the sexual chakra. Lies midway between the pubic bone and belly button. It represents how we express our sexuality and creativity.

Seventh Chakra	Also called the crown chakra. It is situated at the top of head. It represents our connection to the divine.
Sexual Chakra	See Second chakra
Shaman's Death	Spiritual death of the illusion of who you think you are so that you can be reborn in the truth of who you really are.
Sixth Chakra	Also called the third eye. It is situated in the middle of the forehead, above the eyes. It represents intuition and how we see the world.
Solar Plexus	See Third chakra
Soul Path	The path the soul has chosen for its incarnations and learning to achieve full conscious awareness and return to the God source.
Spiritual Body	Our connection to the Divine or God source and holds our spiritual beliefs.
Subconscious Fears	See subconscious resistance
Subconscious Resistance (also called subconscious fears)	Unconscious fear of what will change in their life if they accept change.

Subtle Bodies

The aura is comprised of four major layers: physical body, emotional body, mental body and spiritual body. There are additional subtle bodies such as the astral body and etheric body to name a few.

Theosophy

Is a system of belief based on mystical insight into the nature of God and the soul. It holds that all beliefs attempt to help humanity in evolving to greater perfection, and that each religion therefore has a portion of the truth.

Therapeutic Touch™

Therapeutic touch is an energy-healing system that is gaining prominence in medical facilities and hospitals due to its astounding ability to heal people by the manipulation of energy fields, emotions and feelings. The therapy is based on the belief that the therapist has the capacity to affect the patient's level of pain without prescribing any drugs or even touching the patient physically.

Therapeutic Touch™ was developed by Dolores Krieger, Ph.D., R.N., Professor Emeritus at New York University, and Dora Kunz, a healer. Therapeutic touch takes many of its tenets from visualization, laying on of hands, and aura therapy, three well respected healing practices.

Third Chakra

Also called the solar plexus. It lies between the belly button and the rib cage. It is the chakra of self esteem and represents how safe it is to express ourselves in the world.

Third Eye

An etheric organ of intuitive (psychic) perception that sees beyond the physical world. It is located in the middle of the forehead and is associated with the "brow" or sixth chakra. It is believed to be associated with the pineal gland.

Throat Chakra

See Fifth chakra

Tibetan Medicine

Tibetan medicine is a traditional system of medicine that has been practiced for over 2500 years. It employs a complex approach to diagnosis, incorporating techniques such as pulse analysis and utilizes behavior and dietary modification, medicines composed of natural materials (e.g., herbs and minerals) and physical therapies (e.g. Tibetan acupuncture, moxa-bustion, etc.) to treat illness.

Total Body Modification™ (TBM)

TBM is a technique that combines manual muscle testing with skin reflex points to work with the human bio-computer to locate and correct faulty body energy imbalances that are creating dis-ease. TBM was created in the early 1970s by Victor L. Frank, D.C. when he combined the techniques of master chiropractors, naturopaths, and acupuncturists with the emerging concept of the human bio-computer. For more information: www.tbmseminars.com

Tracking   A term used by healers to describe following the body's stream of consciousness into the core of a blockage.

Trigger   A thought, feeling or belief that elicits an emotional or physical reaction.

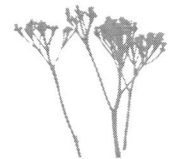

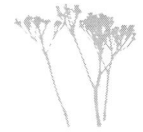

REFERENCES

Adam. (2006). *DreamHealer: A True Story of Miracle Healing.* Canada: Penguin Group (Canada), a division of Pearson Canada Inc.

Andrews, T. (1991). *How to See and Read the Aura.* St. Paul, Minnesota: Llewellyn Publications.

Brennan, B. A. (1987). *Hands of Light.* New York: Ballantine Books.

Dale, C. (2009). *The Subtle Body. An Encyclopoedia of Your Energetic Anatomy.* Boulder, Colorado: Sounds True.

Eden, D. (1999). *Energy Medicine.* New York: Penguin Group.

Ford, D. (1998). *The Dark Side of The Light Chasers.* New York: Riverhead Books.

Hay, L. (2004). *I Can Do It. How To Use Affirmations To Change Your Life.* California: Hay House Inc.

Initiates, T. (1912). *The Kybalion. A Study of The Hermetic Philosophy Of Ancient Egypt and Greece.* Chicago, Ill: The Yogi Publication Society.

Judith, A. P. (2002). *Wheels of Life, A User's Guide To The Chakra System.* St. Paul, Minnesota, USA: Llewellyn Publications.

Magic Eye Inc. & Grossman, M. O. (1993). *Magic Eye. A New Way of Looking at the World.* Kansas City, Mo: Andrews McMeel Publishing.

Tolle, E. (2005). *A New Earth. Awakening to Your Life's Purpose.* United States: Penguin Group.

Virtue, D. P. (1998). *Divine Guidance.* California: Hay House Inc.

Virtue, D. P. (2007). *How to Hear Your Angels.* California: Hay House Inc.

Virtue, D. P. (2001). *The Care and Feeding of Indigo Children.* California: Hay House Inc.

Virture, D. P. (2003). *Archangels & Ascended Masters.* California: Hay House Inc.

Whitfield, C. L. (1987). *Healing the Child Within.* Deerfield Beach, Florida: Health Communications, Inc.

Wilson, L. B. (2005). *de-mystifying...Medical Intuition.* Canada: Lori Wilson Education Corporation.

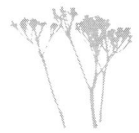

Suggested Reading

Adam. (2006). *DreamHealer: A True Story of Miracle Healing.* Canada: Penguin Group (Canada), a division of Pearson Canada Inc.

Andrews, T. (1991). *How to See and Read the Aura.* St. Paul, Minnesota: Llewellyn Publications.

Ballentine, R. M. (1999). *Radical Healing.* New York: Three Rivers Press.

Brennan, B. A. (1987). *Hands of Light.* New York: Ballantine Books.

Dale, C. (2009). *The Subtle Body. An Encyclopoedia of Your Energetic Anatomy.* Boulder, Colorado: Sounds True.

Eden, D. (1999). *Energy Medicine.* New York: Penguin Group.

Ford, D. (1998). *The Dark Side of The Light Chasers.* New York: Riverhead Books.

Hay, L. (2004). *I Can Do It. How To Use Affirmations To Change Your Life.* California: Hay House Inc.

I. Edward Alcamo, P. (1997). *Anatomy Coloring Workbook.* New York: Random House.

Initiates, T. (1912). T*he Kybalion. A Study of The Hermetic Philosophy Of Ancient Egypt and Greece.* Chicago, Ill: The Yogi Publication Society.

Jampolsky, G. M. (1979). *Love Is Letting Go Of Fear.* Berkeley, California: Celestial Arts.

Judith, A. P. (1996). *Eastern Body, Western Mind.* Berkeley, California: Celestiral Arts Publishing.

Judith, A. P. (2002). *Wheels of Life, A User's Guide To The Chakra System.* St. Paul, Minnesota, USA: Llewellyn Publications.

Krieger, D. P. (1986). *The Therapeutic Touch.* New York: Prentice Hall Press.

Magic Eye Inc. & Grossman, M. O. (1993). *Magic Eye. A New Way of Looking at the World.* Kansas City, Mo: Andrews McMeel Publishing.

Mate, G. M. (2003). *When The Body Says No.* Canada: Alfred. A. Knopf.

Motz, J. (1998). *Hands of Life.* United States: Bantam Books.

Patton, T. (2000). *Structure & Function of the Body.* Mosby Inc.

Ruis, D. M. (1997). *The Four Agreements.* San Rafael, California: Amber-Allen Publishing, Inc.

Salzberg, S. (2002). *Loving-Kindness.* Boston & London: Shambhala.

Tolle, E. (2005). *A New Earth. Awakening to Your Life's Purpose.* United States: Penguin Group.

Virtue, D. P. (1998). *Divine Guidance.* California: Hay House Inc.

Virtue, D. P. (2007). *How to Hear Your Angels.* California: Hay House Inc.

Virtue, D. P. (2001). *The Care and Feeding of Indigo Children.* California: Hay House Inc.

Virture, D. P. (2003). *Archangels & Ascended Masters.* California: Hay House Inc.

Whitfield, C. L. (1987). *Healing the Child Within.* Deerfield Beach, Florida: Health Communications, Inc.

Wilson, L. B. (2005). *de-mystifying...Medical Intuition.* Canada: Lori Wilson Education Corporation.

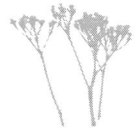

PHOTOGRAPHS

You can order copies of the photographs found in *Following Body Wisdom*. To purchase prints, photocards or other offerings by J. Bruce Walton, please contact him directly at:

www.n8power.com or call directly: 519-766-1250

All transactions for images are the responsibility of the photographer.

SPREAD THE WORD

If this book and its message appeals to you and has helped you with your healing journey, help us spread the word. The following are examples of how you can help.

Give the book to a friend or relative that you believe would benefit from the information.

If you have a website, are on Facebook, Twitter or a blog, consider sharing how you felt about the book and how it helped you on your journey. The more people talk about how energy medicine has helped them and share their stories, the easier it is for others to find the confidence to see if it will help them too.

Write a review and send it to your favourite newspaper, local magazine or newsletter.

If you are an energy medicine practitioner and feel this book will help your clients to understand what you do, put up a display to resell to your clients.

If you know of people in the healing arts or complementary health care field who have a voice to a wider audience, ask them if they would review a copy and make some comments on their website, newsletters or blogs.

The more people who share their story, the greater the impact, the more people are helped. One story can change everything for someone. One voice does make a difference. Go to www.followingbodywisdom.com

"In this life we cannot do great things.
We can only do small things with great love"
Mother Theresa

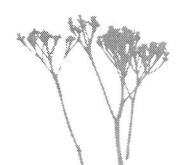